Rania Kaddoussi
Nessrine Fahem

Superior Cave Syndrome and Primary Bronchopulmonary Cancer

Rania Kaddoussi
Nessrine Fahem

Superior Cave Syndrome and Primary Bronchopulmonary Cancer

superior vena cava syndrome

ScienciaScripts

Imprint
Any brand names and product names mentioned in this book are subject to trademark, brand or patent protection and are trademarks or registered trademarks of their respective holders. The use of brand names, product names, common names, trade names, product descriptions etc. even without a particular marking in this work is in no way to be construed to mean that such names may be regarded as unrestricted in respect of trademark and brand protection legislation and could thus be used by anyone.

Cover image: www.ingimage.com

This book is a translation from the original published under ISBN 978-620-6-72256-4.

Publisher:
Sciencia Scripts
is a trademark of
Dodo Books Indian Ocean Ltd. and OmniScriptum S.R.L publishing group

120 High Road, East Finchley, London, N2 9ED, United Kingdom
Str. Armeneasca 28/1, office 1, Chisinau MD-2012, Republic of Moldova, Europe
Printed at: see last page
ISBN: 978-620-8-10211-1

CONTENTS

CHAPTER 1
INTRODUCTION

Superior vena cava syndrome (SVC) is the clinical expression of obstruction of the superior vena cava by extrinsic compression, a process invading the vein or thrombosis. Clinical manifestations are related to the increase in venous pressure upstream of the obstruction and depend on how quickly the obstruction sets in. [1] The first description was made in 1757 by William HUNTER of compression by aortic aneurysm of syphilitic origin. Since then, many aetiologies have been described, and their importance has changed over the years. Whereas in the first half of the twentieth century, infectious diseases were the main causes, malignant mediastinal and pulmonary tumours are now the most common cause of superior vena cava syndrome. It occurs in 3 to 4% of cancer patients, and in 90% of cases is secondary to bronchopulmonary carcinomas and lymphomas.

The clinical picture may be discrete or life-threatening [2]. The aim of this study is to describe the clinical, radiological and evolutionary profile of superior sellar syndrome associated with bronchopulmonary cancer (PBC), as well as the methods of therapeutic management. In this study, we also propose to evaluate the survival of patients with SCS of neoplastic origin and to identify and analyse the various prognostic factors.

CHAPTER 2
MATERIALS AND METHODS

I. Type of study

This is a retrospective study of the records of patients hospitalised in the Pneumology Department at the Fattouma Bourguiba University Hospital in Monastir during the period from 1990 to 2020 for superior cava syndrome secondary to primary bronchopulmonary cancer.

1. Inclusion criteria

- The presence of a clinical or radiological superior vena cava syndrome in patients with histologically confirmed primary bronchial carcinoma of any type.
- Age $\geq$ 18 years.

II. Population study

1. Exclusion criteria

- All cases where the diagnosis has not been confirmed histologically.
- SCS linked to secondary lung cancer.

In all, 108 cases were identified in our study.

III. Collection of data

The information recorded for each patient related to age, sex, occupation, smoking habits, pathological history and respiratory and general functional signs.

The initial assessment included :

- A full physical examination.
- An assessment of body mass index (BMI).
- A chest X-ray
- Bronchial fibroscopy unless contraindicated.
- Means of confirming the diagnosis of PBC
- PBC extension assessment
- Investigations specific to superior vena cava syndrome
- Treatment of CBP and SCS
- PBC and SCS progression and survival.

IV. Classification and assessment

Patients' general condition was assessed using the WHO performance status score (Appendix 1). At the end of the initial work-up, a TNM (Tumor Node Metastasis) classification according to the 7ème edition (appendix 2) was established for each patient.
Evaluation of tumour response to treatment was based on the RECIST

(Response Evaluation Criteria In Solid Tumors) version 1.1 (appendix 3).

V. Survival

This is the length of time between the date of diagnosis of SCS of neoplastic origin and the date of the death or the date of the last news of the patients. Data collection on patient survival was based on medical records for patients who died in hospital and on telephone contact with the family for patients who died at home.

VI. Statistical analysis and study of prognostic factors

The data were entered and analysed using SPSS version 21 software.

Quantitative variables were expressed as means ± standard deviations.
Qualitative variables were expressed as percentages.
Correlations were studied using the X2 test.

Survival was analysed using the Kaplan-Meier method.

Survival was compared according to the different prognostic variables using the Log-Rank test in univariate analysis.
Multivariate analysis was performed using the Cox model to identify independent factors. The model included all variables with a p value < 0.2 in univariate analysis.
For all statistical tests, the statistical significance level was set at 5%.

CHAPTER 3
RESULTS

I. Demographic characteristics of patients

1. Age

The age of our patients at the time of diagnosis ranged from 28 to 88 years, with a mean of 60.2 ± 11.3 years. The majority of patients were aged between 61 and 70 (Figure 1):

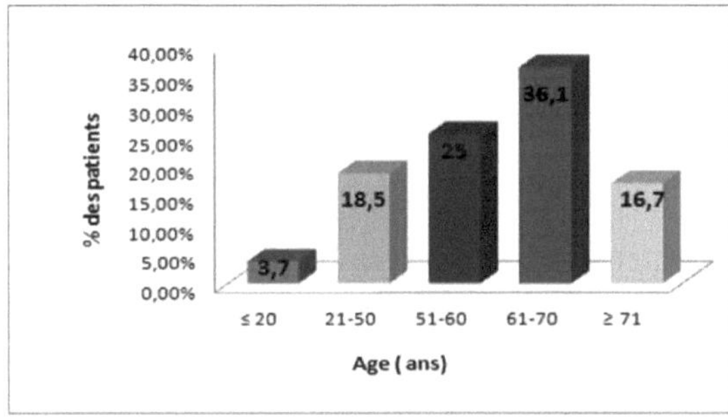

Figure 1: Age distribution of patients

2. Type

The distribution of patients by gender showed a clear male predominance, with 106 men (98%) compared with 2 women (2%) (Figure 2).
The sex ratio was 53.

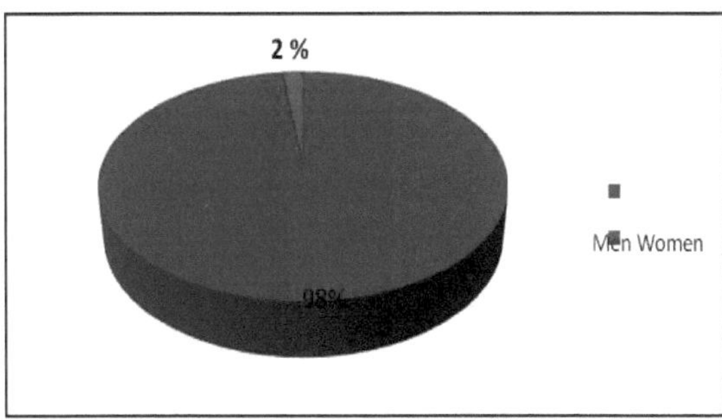

Figure 2: Breakdown of patients by gender

3. Smoking status

Seventy-four patients (68.5%) were smokers and all were male. Smoking ranged from 10 to 132 pack-years (p.a.), with an average of 55.1 p.a. ± 27.2 p.a. (Figure 3).Heavy smoking (≥ 20 PA) was found in 87.7% of smokers. In the 33 ex-smokers, the average duration of smoking cessation was 34.8 months.

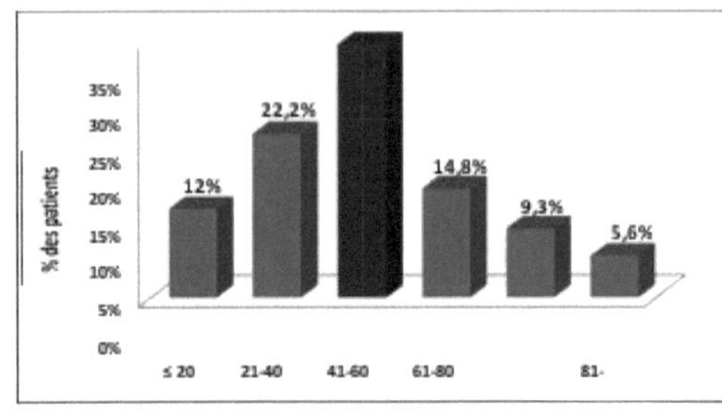

Figure 3: Distribution of patients according to smoking intensity

II. Characteristics clinical

1. Deadline for consultation

The average time elapsed between the appearance of the first functional signs and the first consultation was 59.2 days This delay was greater than 3 months in 25.9% of cases.

2. Clinical

2-1- Manifestations associated with bronchopulmonary cancer 2-1-1- Respiratory signs

Respiratory symptoms consisted mainly of chest pain in 57.4% of cases, cough in 51.8% of cases and dyspnoea of varying intensity in 43.5% of cases. These symptoms were often associated (Figure 4):

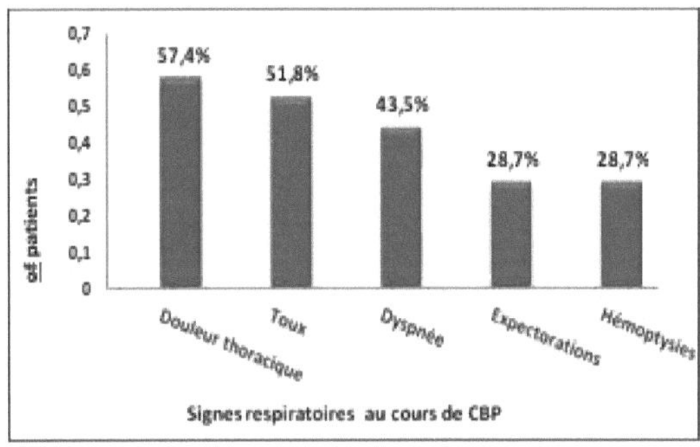

Figure 4: Distribution of respiratory symptoms in bronchopulmonary cancer

2-1-2- Extra-respiratory signs

The main extra-respiratory symptoms are summarised in the following table (table 1):

Table 1: Distribution of extra-respiratory symptoms of bronchopulmonary cancer

Extra-respiratory signs	Number of cases	Percentage (%)
Headaches	4	3,7
Peripheral adenopathy	4	3,7
Motor deficit	3	2,7
Bone pain	2	1,8
Dizziness	2	1,8
Sensory disorders	1	0,9
Abdominal pain	1	0,9
Dysphonia	9	8,3
Dysphagia	2	1,8

Metastases were indicative of PBC in 19 patients (15.4%). The most frequent secondary sites were the brain in 3 cases (2.8%) and lymph nodes in 4 cases (3.7%).

2-1-3- General signs

Changes in general condition were noted in 35 patients (32.4%), with asthenia, anorexia and weight loss. Weight loss varied between 1 and 26 kg, with an average of 8.1±5.5 kg.

2-1-4- Incidental discoveries

Incidental radiological discovery of PBC was noted in 6 patients (5.5%).

2-1-5- Physical signs

- **WHO Performance Status Score (PS) :**

Assessment of general condition at the time of diagnosis of PBC according to the WHO PS score revealed a PS ≤ 2 in 24 patients (22.2%) (Table 2) :

Table 2: WHO Performance Status Score (PS)

	PS		Number of cases	Percentage (%)
0		7		6,48
1		77		71,2
≥ 2		24		22,2

- **Chest signs :**

Physical examination of the lungs revealed polypnoea in 31 patients (28.7%), pleural fluid syndrome in 11 patients (10.1%) and superior venous syndrome in 63 patients (58.3%). The examination was normal in 45 patients (41%).

- **Extra-thoracic signs :**

Digital hippocratism was noted in 14 patients (12.9%), peripheral adenopathy (cervical, supra-clavicular and axillary) in 21 patients (19.4%), fever in 5 patients and a skin nodule in 4 patients. The neurological examination showed a motor deficit in 5 cases (4.6%), paresthesias in 2 cases (1.8%) and a cerebellar syndrome in 1 case (table 3):

Table 3: Extra-thoracic signs of bronchopulmonary cancer

Extra-thoracic signs		Number of cases		Percentage (%)
Peripheral adenopathy	21		19,4	
Digital hippocratism	14		12,9	
Fever	5		4,6	
Skin nodule	4		3,7	
Hepatomegaly	3		2,7	
Motor deficit	5		4,6	
Paresthesias	2		1,8	
Cerebellar syndrome	1		0,9	

2-2- Clinical manifestations specific to superior cava syndrome

In the group studied, superior vena cava obstruction was symptomatic in 63 patients (58.3%), and radiologically detectable in the remainder. Superior vena cava syndrome was indicative of PBC in 45 patients (41.7%). It was metachronous (appeared after the discovery of PBC) in 18 cases (16.6%) of the patients with an average onset of 30 days.

• Clinical signs suggestive of SCS :

In addition to functional respiratory signs suggestive of SCS, such as dyspnoea or cough, and neurological signs such as headaches in 4 of our patients and dizziness in 2 patients, haemodynamic signs specific to SCS were noted in 63 patients, and these signs were often associated. Filling of the supra-clavicular recesses and facial oedema were the most frequent signs (table 4):

Table 4: Physical signs of superior vena cava syndrome

Physical signs of DBS	Number of cases	Percentage (%)
Facial oedema	43	68,2
Filling of the supra-clavicular recesses	49	77,7
Collateral venous circulation	39	61,9
Increased neck volume	26	41,2
Turgidity of the jugular veins	24	38
Cyanosis	5	7,9
Oedema of the upper limbs	13	20,6

• Gasometry :

Room air blood gases were measured in 67 patients (62%). Hypoxaemia ≤ 70mmHg was noted in 21 patients (19.4%) with severe hypoxaemia ≤ 55mmHg in 6 patients (5.6%). Hypercapnia was noted in 4 patients (3.7%).

• Signs of seriousness :

Clinical and gasometric signs of severity were noted in 8 patients. Inspiratory dyspnoea was the predominant sign (table 5):

Table 5: Signs of severity of superior vena cava syndrome

Signs of seriousness	Number	Percentage (%)
Dyspnoea	6	9.5
Desaturation	6	9.5
Cyanosis	5	7.9
Signs of struggle	5	7.9

III. Chest X-ray

Chest X-rays were taken in all patients. The various radiological aspects are summarised in the table below (Table 6):

Table 6: Radiological aspects of bronchopulmonary cancer

Radiological aspects	Number of cases	Percentage (%)
Normal	1	0 ,9
Hilar opacities	36	33,3
Mediastino-pulmonary opacities	27	25
Intra-parenchymal opacities	22	20,3
Mediastinal enlargement	13	12
Infiltrate	2	1,8
White lung	3	2,7
Costal lysis	1	0,9

The topography of the opacities was predominantly right in 92 patients (85.2%).

IV. Fibroscopy bronchial

Tracheobronchial fibroscopy was performed in 94 patients (87%). Fibroscopy was contraindicated in 10 cases (9.2%) and refused by 4 patients (3.7%). Pathology was detected in 85 patients (90.4%). The various endoscopic aspects are shown in the following table (Table 7):

Table 7: Endoscopic aspects of bronchopulmonary cancer

Endoscopic aspects		Number	Percentage (%)
Endobronchial stenosis	40		37
Infiltration of the mucosa	35		32,4
bronchial			
Thickening of the spurs	41	40	
Endoluminal bud	30	27,7	
Inflammation	13	12	
Intrinsic compression	12	11,1	
Bleeding	3	2,7	
Paralysis of the vocal cords.	3	2,7	
Normal	9	8,3	

The location of endoscopic lesions is detailed in the following table (Table 8):

Table 8: Location of endoscopic lesions in bronchopulmonary cancer

Headquarters		Workforce		Percentage (%)
Trachea	16		18,8	
Carene	12		14,1	
Right main bronchus	22		25,8	
Left main bronchus	7		8,23	
Upper right lobar	57		67	
Middle right lobar	6		7	
Lower right lobar	7		8,2	
Intermediate trunk	16		18,8	

Bronchial biopsies were taken in 64 cases, i.e. 68% of the fibroscopies performed.

V. Confirmation of diagnosis

Confirmation of the diagnosis was obtained by various means, which are summarised in the following table (table 9):

Table 9: Means of confirming the diagnosis

Means of confirming the diagnosis	Number of cases	Percentage (%)
Bronchial biopsy	64	59,2
Cytology of bronchial fluid	7	6,4
Tumour biopsy under CT scan	19	17,5
Thoracotomy	4	3,7
Pleural biopsy	3	2,7
Cytology of pleural fluid	1	0,9
Sputum cytology	1	0,9
Biopsy of peripheral adenopathy	5	4,6
Skin biopsy	3	2,7
Biopsy of a metastasis	2	1,8
Cytopuncture of lymph nodes	7	6,4

VI. Anatomopathology

Histopathological confirmation was carried out in all patients. The anatomopathological study of the various samples showed : Small cell carcinoma (SCC) in 40.7% of cases, squamous cell carcinoma (SCC) in 29.6% of cases and adenocarcinoma (ADK) in 25.9% of cases. The different histological types are grouped together in the following figure (Figure 5):

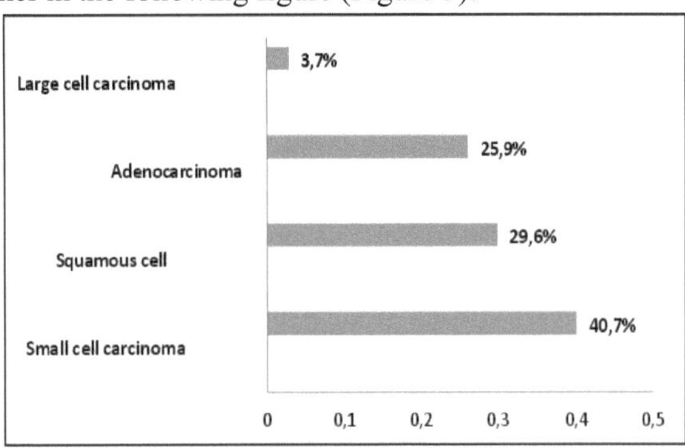

Figure 5: Distribution of histological types of bronchopulmonary cancer

VII. Investigation of superior vena cava syndrome and assessment of extension

1. Chest computed tomography (CT)

1-1- Investigation of superior cave syndrome

Chest CT with contrast injection was used to diagnose obstruction of the superior vena cava in 106 patients, i.e. in 98.1% of cases; two patients died before chest CT was performed. The time taken to perform a CT scan in symptomatic patients in relation to the clinical signs of DBS ranged from 3 days to 77 days, with an average of 28 days. This examination also made it possible to diagnose DBS in 45 asymptomatic patients. Chest CT showed tumour invasion in 62.2% of cases, extrinsic compression of the SVC in 37.7% of cases, which was mainly due to the tumour, and collateral venous circulation in 17.9% of cases. The different types of damage found on thoracic CT scans are summarised in the following figure (Figure 6):

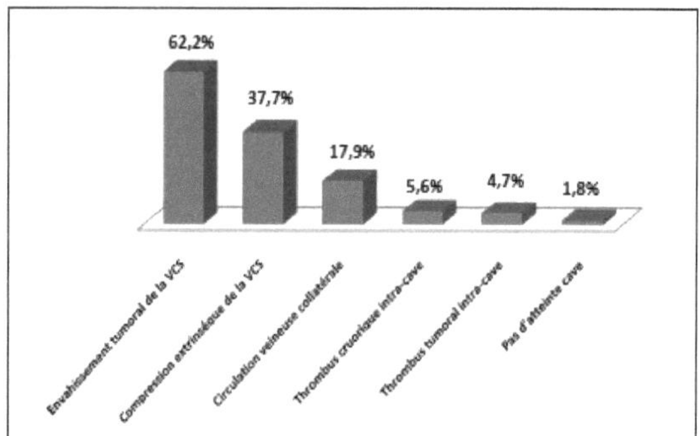

Figure 6: Scans of superior vena cava syndrome

1-2- Locoregional invasion and metastases

Locoregional invasion occurred mainly in the vena cava. in 98.1% of cases, the pulmonary artery in 43.3% of cases, the trachea in 30.1% of cases, the parietal pleura in 30.1% of cases and the aorta in 20.7% of cases (figure 7).

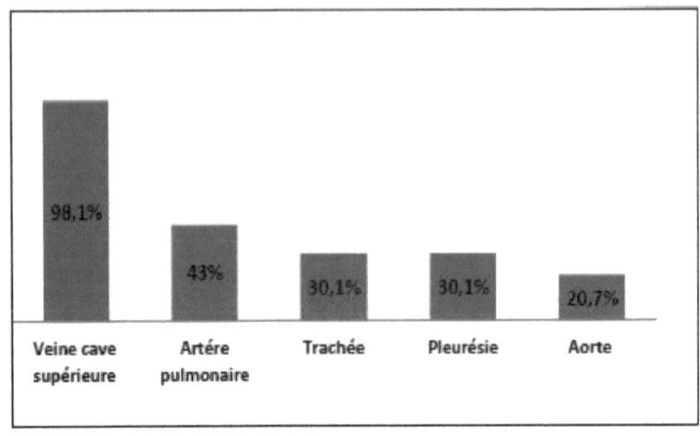

Figure 7: Chest CT scan: Locoregional invasion

Homolateral pulmonary localisations were found in 11 patients (15.2%) and contralateral in 20 patients (27.7%).

2. Ultrasound abdominal

Abdominal ultrasound was performed in 63 patients, 50 of whom returned normal. The secondary abdominal locations most frequently found were hepatic in 8 patients and adrenal in 5 patients. The various metastases are detailed in the following table (table 10):

Table 10: Secondary locations of bronchopulmonary cancer on abdominal ultrasound.

Metastases	Number of employees (n)		Percentage (%)
Single hepatic		1	1,5
Multiple liver disease		5	7,9
Unilateral adrenal		3	4,7
Bilateral adrenal		1	1,5
Isolated abdominal adenopathy		1	1,5

3. Cerebral CT

Cerebral CT scans were performed in 78 patients, 68 of whom were normal. Cerebral metastases were found in 7 patients and cerebral metastases associated with cerebellar metastases in 3 patients.

4. Other investigations for superior vena cava syndrome 4-1- Cervical ultrasound

Cervical ultrasound was performed in 8 of our patients. Jugular thrombosis was found in 2 patients, jugular thrombosis associated with subclavian thrombosis in 1 patient, jugular thrombosis associated with cervical adenopathy in 1 patient and isolated cervical adenopathy in 1 patient, the rest of the patients had normal cervical ultrasound.

4-2- Venous Doppler ultrasound of the upper limbs

Upper limb venous Doppler ultrasound was performed in 5 patients. It showed thrombosis in 2 cases: one subclavian and the other subclavian. radial, ulnar and subclavian.

VIII. Stadiums

1. Small cell carcinoma (SCC)

The CPC was in the diffuse stage in 28.7% of cases (Table 11).

Table 11: Classification of small cell cancer

Stadiums	Number of cases	Percentage (%)
Located	13	12
Broadcast	31	28,7
Total	44	40,7

2. Non-small cell carcinoma (NSCC)

NSCLC was diagnosed at an advanced stage in 35 patients, i.e. in 32.4% of cases (Table 12).

Table 12: Classification of non-small cell cancer

Stadiums	Number		Percentage (%)
IIIA		10	9,2
IIIB		19	17,6
IV		35	32,4
Total		64	59,2

IX. Treatment

Patients were managed in 2 ways: symptomatic treatment of superior vena cava syndrome and management of PBC.

1. Symptomatic treatment of superior cava syndrome

In the group of patients studied, the symptomatic treatment of SCS involved a combination of oxygen therapy, corticosteroids, anti-coagulants and diuretics. Depressive thoracic radiotherapy was used in some patients.

1-1- Treatment

The time between discovery of DBS and drug treatment ranged from 3 to 150 days, with an average of 25.3 days.

1-1-1- Oxygen therapy

Oxygen therapy was administered in 15 patients (13.4%). The flow rate varied from 1 to 6 l/min. Long-term oxygen therapy (LTO) was indicated in 4 patients with hypoxaemia $\leq$ 55 mmHg.

1-1-2- Corticosteroid therapy

Corticosteroids were administered in 63 patients (58.3%). Initial parenteral corticosteroid therapy was based essentially on hydrocortisone hemisuccinate (HCS) at a dose of 200 to 800 mg/d.Follow-up oral corticosteroid therapy was based on Prednisolone at a dose of 10 to 120mg/d in 75% of patients. Sodium restriction was associated in all cases. The average duration of intravenous treatment was 14.5 $\pm$ 9 days. The total duration of corticosteroid therapy ranged from 12 to 192 days with an average of 81.3 $\pm$ 68.7 days.

1-1-3- Anti-coagulation

Anti-coagulation was administered in 30 patients (27.7%). Low molecular weight heparin (LMWH) in curative dose was used in 27 patients and unfractionated heparin in 3 patients. Overlapping anti-coagulation used anti-vitamin K in 7 patients and the others kept the LMWH. The total duration of anticoagulant treatment ranged from 5 to 144 days, with an average of 14 days.

1-1-4- Diuretics

Diuretics were prescribed in only 1 patient.

1-2- Thoracic radiotherapy decompressive

Forty-two patients (38.8%) underwent depressive thoracic radiotherapy.
High-dose rapid external mediastino-pulmonary irradiation was performed at a dose of 3 Grays per day for the first few days, with a total dose of 6 to 30 Grays.

The average time between superior vena cava syndrome and de-compressive thoracic radiotherapy was estimated at 40 days.

2. Management of bronchopulmonary cancer

2-1- Symptomatic treatment

Symptomatic treatment was prescribed in 106 patients (98.1%) (table13) :

Table 13: Symptomatic treatments for bronchopulmonary cancer.

Treatment	Number of cases	Percentage (%)
Minor painkillers	55	51,8
Morphine analgesics	50	47,1
Corticoids	63	59,4
Long-term oxygen therapy	4	3,7
Anticoagulants	30	28,3
Thoracic decompressive radiotherapy	42	39,6
Decompressive spinal cord radiotherapy	2	1,8
Palliative cerebral radiotherapy	9	8,4

2-2- Curative thoracic radiotherapy

Twenty-seven patients (25%) underwent curative thoracic radiotherapy. The curative RT dose varied from 20 grays to 65 grays and the mean dose was 38 ± 18.4 grays. The mean time from diagnosis of PBC to radiotherapy was 113.3 ± 62.1 days.

2-3- Chemotherapy

2-3-1- First-line chemotherapy

Chemotherapy was indicated in 82 patients (76%). The main contraindications to chemotherapy were impairment of general condition (18 cases), advanced age (1 case), respiratory failure (4 cases), infectious aetiology (2 cases) or refusal by the patient (1 case). The mean time from diagnosis to chemotherapy was 40 days. The mean number of courses was 4.1 ± 2.5. Fifty-five patients (51%) received at least 3 courses of chemotherapy.A combination of two products was used in almost all patients.

► **CNPC :**

Table 14: First-line chemotherapy according to stage in NSCLC

Stades	*Nombre des cas*	*Pourcentage (%)*
IIIA	4	4 ,8
IIIB	16	19,5
IV	26	31,7

The first-line chemotherapy products used are summarised in the table below (table 15):

Table 15: First-line chemotherapy products for NSCLC

Type of association	Number of cases	
Alimta		1
Cisplatyl-VP16		12
Cisplatyl-Gemzar		13
Cisplatyl-Taxotere		2
Cisplatyl-Alimta		9
Carboplatin-Gemzar		2
Carboplatin-Navelbine		1

► **CPC :**

The chemotherapy prescribed was based on VP16 and platinum salts.

Table 16: Chemotherapy in CPC

Classification	Number of cases		Percentage (%)
Located		13	15,8
Broadcast		26	31,7

The first-line chemotherapy products used are summarised in the following table (table 17):

Table 17: First-line chemotherapy products in CPC

Type d'association	*Nombre des cas*
Cisplatyl-VP16	37
Carboplatine-VP16	2

2-3-2- Second-line chemotherapy

Five patients received second-line chemotherapy after failing to respond to first-line chemotherapy.The number of treatments was 2.33±0.8. The products used are summarised in the following table (table 18):

Table 18: Second-line chemotherapy

CNPC		CPC	
Cisplatyl-Taxotére	1		
Taxotére	1	Cisplatyl-VP16	2
Cisplatyl-Gemzar	1		

3. Treatment-related complications 3-1- Drug treatment

Hyponatremia complicated only one case treated with corticosteroids for superior cava syndrome.

3-2- Radiotherapy (RT) thoracic

Complications related to RT occurred in 18 cases, including 7 patients who developed a radiodermatitis and 8 patients had post-radiation oesophagitis (table 19):

Table 19: Complications of thoracic radiotherapy in bronchopulmonary cancer and superior vena cava syndrome

Type of complication	Workforce	
Radiodermatitis		7
Esophagitis		8
Fibrosis		1
Candidiasis		1
Laryngitis		1

3-3- Chemotherapy

The main complications of chemotherapy were haematological in 28 patients, digestive in 25 and hepatic in 9. The following table details the complications found (table 20):

Table 20: Complications of chemotherapy

Type of complication Nature de Number Percentage complication		
Anemia	17	30,35%
Haematological toxicity Leukopenia	11	19,64%
Neutropenia	10	17,85%
Thrombocytopenia	6	10,71%
Digestive toxicity vomiting	24	42,85%
diarrhoea	1	1,7%
Liver toxicity cytolysis	4	7,1%
Cholestasis	5	8,9%
Renal toxicity	2	3,5%
Alopecia	3	5,3%

X. Evolution

1. Superior vena cava syndrome

1-1- Response to treatment

The response of SCS to treatment was assessed in 69 patients. The time taken to respond to treatment ranged from 10 to 60 days, with a mean of 29 days. ± 18.1 days.

► Clinically, 50 patients were re-evaluated: 9 patients presented a complete response, 29 patients showed a partial response, 9 patients showed worsening of the SCS and 2 patients showed stabilisation.

► In terms of scans, 14 patients were re-evaluated, 11 of whom showed regression of tumour invasion of the SVC.

► Only 5 patients were clinically and scannographically assessed. The time between the SCS and the evaluation scan ranged from 7 days to 168 days, with an average of 104 ± 44.7 days.

Table 21: Different types of response to treatment in superior vena cava syndrome

Type of response NumberNature of response Number percentage			
Full answer		11	16%
Clinical response55Partial response		32	46 ,3%
Worsening of SCS		9	13%
stabilisation		3	4 ,3%
Regression of			
Response invasion		15	21,7%
scans	tumour syndrome		
19	upper cellar		
	Waterproofing of		
	the vena cava	4	5,7%
	superior		

The response of superior vena cava syndrome to drug treatment is detailed in the following table (table 22):

Table 22: Response of SCS to drug treatment.

	Réponse complète	*Réponse partielle*	*Stabilisation*	*Aggravation*
Corticoïdes	7	15	0	5
Corticoïdes + Anticoagulants	2	13	2	3

The response of superior vena cava syndrome to thoracic decompressive radiotherapy was noted in 28 patients (table23):

Table 23: SCS response to thoracic decompressive radiotherapy.

	Réponse complète	*Réponse partielle*	*Stabilisation*	*Aggravation*
Radiothérapie thoracique décompressive	7	21	2	4

1-2- Recidivism

Recurrence of SCS after initial clinical or scannographic improvement was noted in 12 patients, i.e. in 11.1% of cases. It was essentially clinical in 11 patients with an average delay of 22 days.

❖ Of these 12 patients: 5 had a recurrence of superior venous cava syndrome on drug treatment, 3 undergoing chemotherapy and 2 undergoing a combination of medical treatment and chemotherapy, and 2 undergoing thoracic decompressive radiotherapy.
The treatment of this recurrence involved several methods, which are summarised in the table below (table24):

Table 24: Treatment of recurrence in superior vena cava syndrome

Medium	Workforce		Percentage (%)	
Corticoids		12		100
LMWH curative dose		6		50
HNF		1		8,3
O2		4		33,3
Palliative RT		6		50

2. Broncho- lung cancer

2-1- Response to chemotherapy

Of the 82 patients who received chemotherapy, 45 were evaluated (Table 25):

Table 25: Response to chemotherapy in PBC

	CPC		CNPC
Total response		1	1
Partial response		20	7
Stabilisation		2	4
Tumour progression		4	6

2-2- Response to curative thoracic radiotherapy

27 patients underwent curative thoracic radiotherapy, with response assessed in 9 patients (table 26):

Table 26: Response to curative thoracic radiotherapy in SCS and CBP

	CPC		CNPC
Total response		3	3
Partial response		1	0
No answer		1	1

XI. Survival and prognostic factors

1. Survival overall

Eighty-nine patients (82.4%) died, 9 patients (8.3%) survived and 10 patients were lost to follow-up. The median survival of our patients was 7 months. Survival at 1 and 2 years was 22% and 6% respectively.

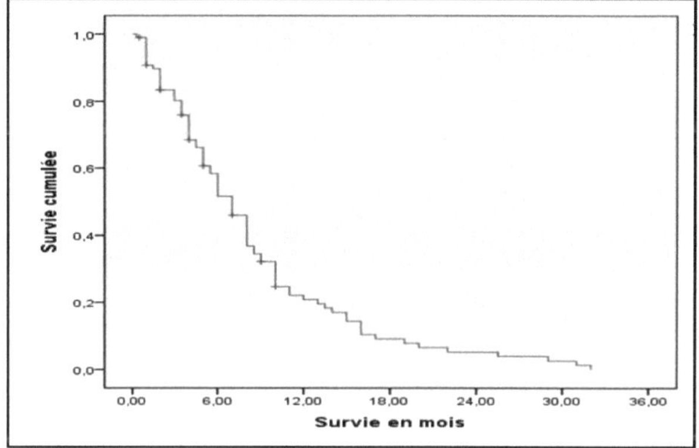

Figure 8: Overall survival curve

2. Prognostic factors

A. Study univariate

1. Characteristics demographics

1-1- Age

Patients aged over 60 had a greater survival rate than patients aged under 60, but the difference was statistically insignificant (table 27).

Table 27: Survival as a function of age

Age	Nombre des cas	Médiane de survie en mois	P
≤ 60 ans	46	6 ±1,07	
< 60 ans	52	7 ± 0,81	0,22

1-2- Sex

Men had better survival than women, but the difference was statistically insignificant (table 28):

Table 28: Survival by sex

Gender	Number of cases	Median survival	P
Men	97	7 ± 0,60	0,14
Women	1	3,5 ± 0,60	

1-3- Smoking

1-3-1- Smoking status

Non-smokers and ex-smokers had a higher survival rate than smokers, but the difference was statistically insignificant (table 29):

Table 29: Survival according to smoking status

Smoking status	Number of cases	Median survival in months	P
Non-smokers or ex-smokers	33	8 ± 1,57	0,13
Smokers	65	6 ± 0,69	

1-3-2- Smoking

Among smokers and ex-smokers, there was no statistically significant difference between patients in terms of smoking habits (table 30):

Table 30: Survival according to smoking habits

Smoking habits Number of cases Median de survival P en month		
≤ 50 PA	53	7 ± 0,872 0,35
> 50 PA	45	7 ± 0,762
2. Clinical characteristics		

2-1- Respiratory co-morbidities

Median survival was close between patients with and without respiratory co-morbidities, but the difference was not significant (table31):

Table 31: Survival according to respiratory co-morbidities

Co-morbiditiesNumber of casesMedian survival in monthsP respiratory			
no	66	7 ± 0,93	0,5
yes	32	7 ± 1,05	

2-2- BMI

Obese patients survived longer than the rest of the patients, but the difference was statistically insignificant (table 32):

Table 32: Survival as a function of BMI

BMINumber of cases		Median survival in months	P	
<18,5	10	6 ± 3,55		
18,5-24,99	44	7 ± 0,68		0,07
≥25	15	10± 5,87		
2-3- Co-wasting				

Median survival was almost the same for patients with recent weight loss and those without, and the difference was not statistically significant (table 33):

Table 33: Survival according to weight loss

Weight loss Number	Survival median in months P		
no	83	7 ± 0,671	0,18
yes	15	7 ± 2,714	
2-4- General condition			

General condition, as assessed by the WHO performance status score, clearly influenced the survival of our patients. Indeed, the median survival of patients with a WHO PS score < 2 was 8 months compared with 3.5 months for patients with a score ≥2 with a statistically significant difference (table 34) (figure 10):

Table 34: Survival according to WHO PS score

WHO PS score		Number of casesSurvival medianP			
<	2	75	8 ± 0,60	< 0,001	
≥	2	23	3.5 ± 0,79		

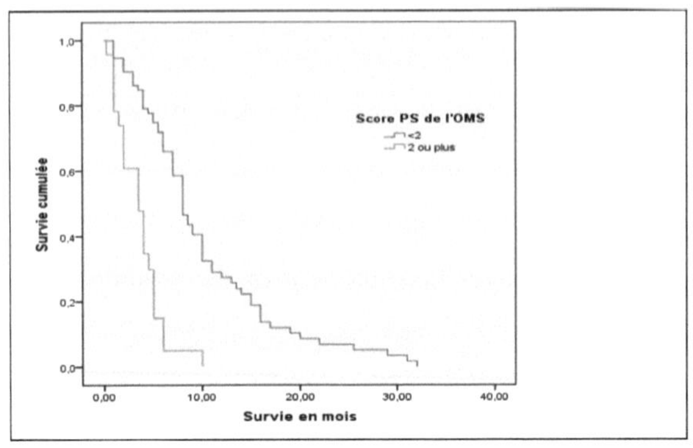

Figure 9: Survival curve as a function of WHO PS score.

3. Respiratory function characteristics 3-1- FEV1

Patients with FEV1 ≥ 70% of the theoretical value had a better survival compared to patients with a ventilatory deficit with FEV1 < 70 %. The difference was statistically significant (Table 35) (Figure 9):

Table 35: Survival as a function of FEV1

FEV1	Number of cases	Median survival in months	p
< 70%	48	6 ± 0,83	0,04
≥70%	23	9 ± 1	

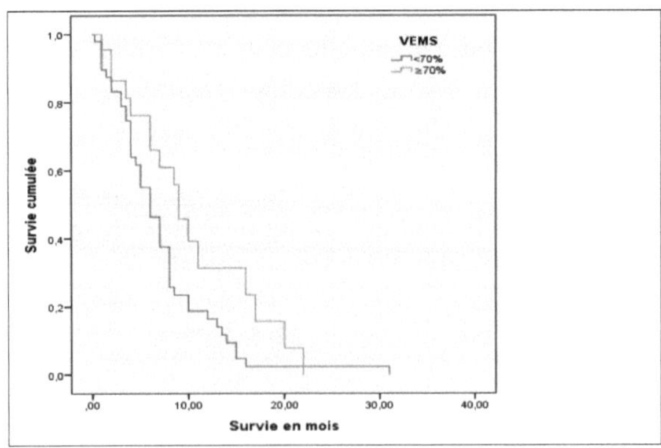

Figure 10: Survival curve as a function of FEV1.

3-2- PaO2

Chronic respiratory failure significantly reduced the survival of our patients. patients (table36) (figure 10):

Table 36: Survival as a function of PaO2

PaO2	Nombre de cas	Médiane de survie en mois	P
< 70 mmHg	17	4 ± 0,5	0,017
≥ 70 mmHg	62	8 ± 0,74	

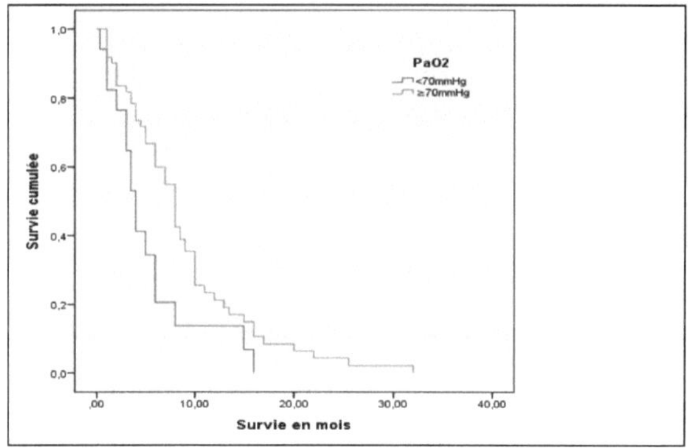

Figure 11: Survival curve as a function of PaO2.

3-3- PaCO2

Hypercapnia reduced patient survival but the difference was not statistically significant. significant (table 37):

Table 37: Survival as a function of PaCO2

PaCO2	Number of cases	Median survival in months	P
< 45 mmHg	75	7 ± 0,8	0,5
≥ 45 mmHg	2	6	

4. Anatomopathology and extension assessment

4-1- Histological type

The survival of patients with small cell carcinoma was better than those with non-small cell carcinoma, with a statistically significant difference (table 38) (figure 11):

Table 38: Survival by histological type

Type histological	Number of cases	Median survival in months	P
CNPC	61	5 ± 0,60	
CPC	37	8.5 ± 0,94	0,002

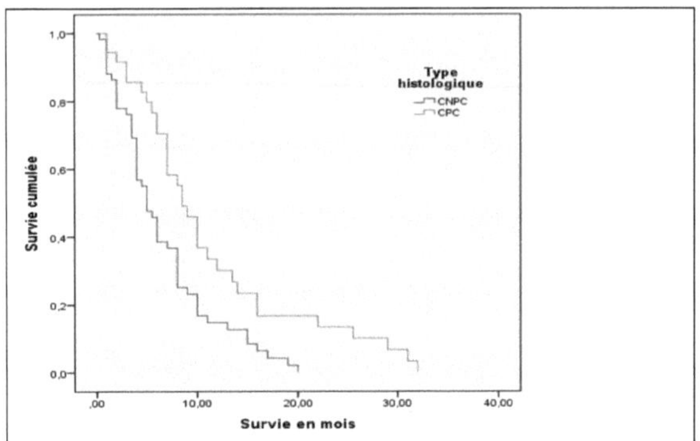

Figure 12: Survival curve according to histological type

4-2- Assessment of extension

4-2-1- TNM stages

- **CNPC :**

Patients with localised or locally advanced tumours had better survival than those with metastatic tumours, but the difference was not statistically significant (table 39).

Table 39: Survival by stage of NSCLC

Stadium	Number of cases	Median survival in months	P	
IIIA	8	6 ± 1,41		
IIIB	11	9 ± 1,8		0,13
IV	42	5 ± 0,4		

- **CPC :**

Patients with diffuse tumours had reduced survival (table 40):

Table 40: Survival according to stage of CPC

Stadium	Number of cases	Median survival in months	P
located	11	13 ± 2,37	0,11
Broadcast	26	7 ± 1,04	

4-2-2- Number of metastatic sites

Patients with a single metastatic site had better survival than patients with multiple metastatic sites, with a statistically significant difference (table 41) (figure 12):

Table 41: Survival as a function of the number of metastatic sites

Number of sites metastatic	Number of cases	Median survival in month	p
1	27	7 ± 0,94	0,061
≥ 2	40	5 ± 0,72	

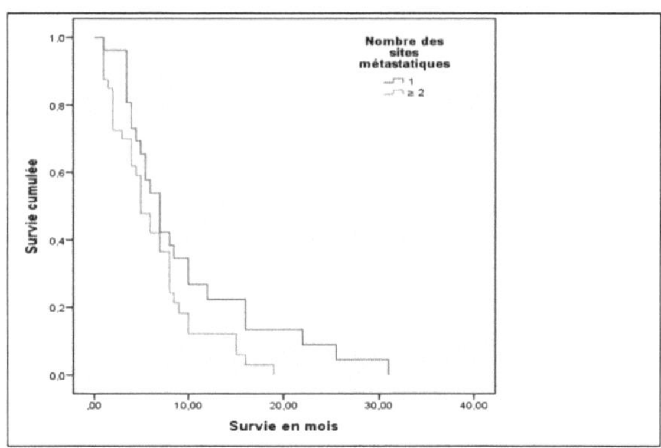

Figure 13: Survival curve as a function of the number of metastatic sites

5. Superior cava syndrome

5-1- Symptomatic versus non-symptomatic superior venous syndrome

Survival was better in non-symptomatic patients but the statistical difference was not significant (table 42):

Table 42: Survival according to DBS symptomatology

Superior vena cava syndrome symptomatic	Number of case	Median survival in months	P
No	44	8 ± 0,51	
Yes	54	5.5 ± 0,65	0,19

5-2- Signs of the severity of the superior cava syndrome

Patients with DBS with signs of severity had a shorter survival with a statistically significant difference (table 43) (figure 13) :

Table 43: Survival according to signs of DBS severity

Signs of gravity	Number of cases	Median survival in months	P
no	87	7 ±0,57	
yes	6	3 ± 91	0,028

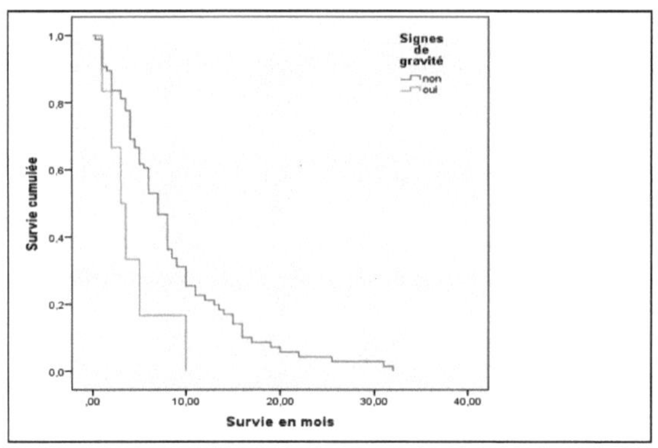

Figure 14: Survival curve according to signs of DBS severity

6. Treatment

6-1- Treatment of bronchopulmonary cancer

6-1-1- Treatment of NSCLC

Patients treated with chemotherapy alone had better survival in our series than other patients treated with radiotherapy, radio-chemotherapy or symptomatic treatment alone (table44) (figure14) :

Table 44: Survival of NSCLC according to treatment

Treatment	Number of cases	Median survival in months	P
Symptomatic treatment	19	4 ± 1,06	0,003
Curative radiotherapy	5	4 ± 0,27	
Chemotherapy	25	8 ± 0,47	
Radiochemotherapy	12	4 ± 0,52	

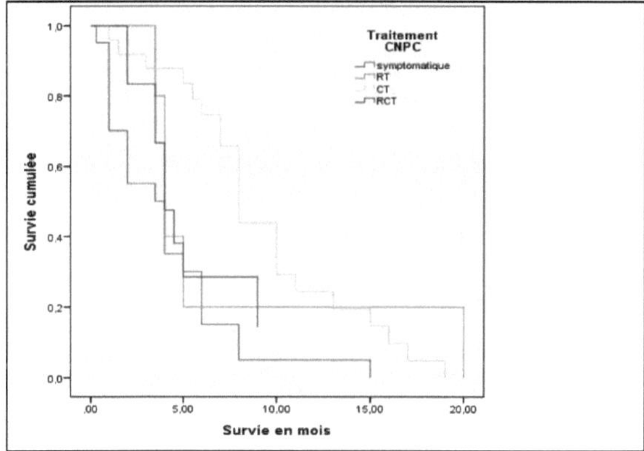

Figure 15: Survival curve for NSCLC as a function of treatment

6-1-2- Treatment of CPC

Patients treated with radio-chemotherapy had a better survival (table 45) (figure 15) :

Table 45: Survival of CPCs according to treatment

Treatment	Number of cases	Median survival in months	P
Symptomatic treatment	3	3	< 0,001
Radiochemotherapy	5	29 ± 11	
Chemotherapy	29	8,5 ± 1,28	

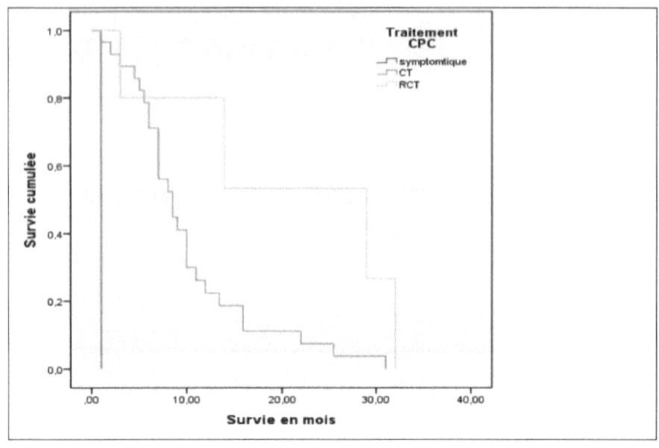

Figure 16: Survival curve for CPC as a function of treatment

6-2- Treatment of superior cave syndrome

6-2-1- Decompressive thoracic radiotherapy

Patients who received decompressive thoracic RT had better survival than those who did not receive palliative thoracic RT (table46).

Table 46: Survival according to thoracic decompressive RT :

Thoracic radiotherapy decompressive	Number of cases	Median survival in months	P
Not done	17	4 ± 1,02	0,15
Made	37	6 ± 1,43	

6-2-2- Treatment

Drug treatment of SCS had an influence on patient survival, but the difference was not significant (table47) (figure 16):

Table 47: Survival according to SCS drug treatment

Drug treatment of superior vena cava syndrome	Number case	fro m	Median survival in months	P
No	61	6 ± 0,95		0,6
Yes	31	8 ± 0,83		

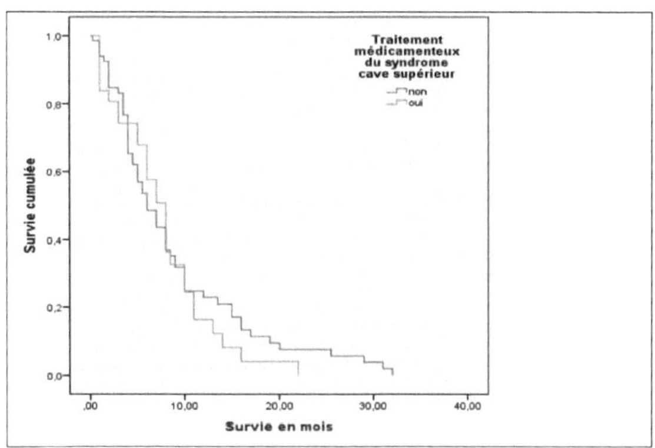

Figure 17: Survival curve as a function of drug treatment for DBS

B. Multi- study

Factors predictive of mortality from superior vena cava syndrome in PBC were : Male sex, smoking status, deterioration in general condition, presence of 2 metastases or more and the presence of clinical signs of DBS severity.

Table 48: Multivariate study of factors predicting mortality from superior vena cava syndrome in PBC

	HR	95% CI	P
Male sex	13,78	1,7-111,9	0,014
Smoking status	1,78	1,1-2,9	0.019
Impaired general condition	5,28	2,9-9,5	< 0,001
Metastases > 2	2,26	1,2-4,3	0,12
Signs of seriousness	2,59	1,08-6,17	0,03

CHAPTER 4
DISCUSSION

Superior vena cava syndrome (SVC), associated with obstruction of the superior vena cava (SVC) and/or brachiocephalic venous trunks, was first described by William Hunter in 1757, based on the observation of a patient with a saccular aneurysm of the thoracic aorta complicating tertiary syphilis [3]. In 1857, William Stockes described an even more serious condition in a 36-year-old man with oedema of the neck and face, extreme dyspnoea and dilatation of the right jugular vein and superficial thoraco-abdominal veins [4].

Obstruction of the CSV may be acute or chronic, partial or total. It may result from extrinsic compression, infiltration of the venous wall by a tumour or, more rarely, thrombosis. While the proportion of non-tumour etiologies is tending to increase, particularly as a result of the increasingly frequent use of central venous catheters, SCS remains predominantly associated with a malignant lesion in 74% to 95% of cases [2,5,6,7,8,9,10,11]. Today, bronchopulmonary cancer accounts for 80 to 85% of the most frequent causes of SCS in adults [9, 10, 12, 13, 14,15]. Through this study, we have tried to draw up a demographic, clinical, radiological and evolutionary profile, as well as the therapeutic management of the superior vena cava syndrome linked to bronchopulmonary cancer. We also tried to determine the survival of patients with SCS of malignant origin as well as the main prognostic factors.

1. Anatomical-physiopathological background

Superior vena cava syndrome (SVC) is the clinical expression of obstruction of the superior vena cava (SVC) by extrinsic compression, most commonly a process invading the vein or thrombosis leading to increased venous pressure in the encephalic, brachial and thoracic territories. As a component of Barety's compartment, the SCV is the structure in this restricted space that offers the least resistance to compression due to its thin wall and the low pressure (< 5 mmHg) within it. In tumour pathology, SCS is most often secondary to compression. extrinsic by a mass of the middle and/or anterior mediastinum, in particular a tumour of the right upper lobe or paratracheal or precarenal adenopathies. Following this compression, collateral circulation develops to divert blood flow towards the azygos system or the inferior vena cava and then the heart. The main bypass routes are represented by the azygos vein, the internal mammary vein, the lateral thoracic veins, the spinal plexuses, and the thoraco-epigastric, phrenic and mediastinal veins.This venous circulation will develop progressively, in most cases leading to a reduction in venous blood pressure and a state of equilibrium. An acute SCS will therefore be much more difficult to tolerate than a chronically evolving cava syndrome, in which case the collaterals will have had time to develop. The progression of malignant SCS is usually rapid, with an average of 3.2 weeks elapsing between the onset of SCS and its diagnosis. Other factors influence the severity and tolerability of superior vena cava syndrome, in particular the level of obstruction in relation to the azygos vein outlet, with clinical symptoms being all the more marked if the obstruction is located below the azygos vein outlet. Other factors involved in the tolerance of SCS are the degree of obstruction of the superior vena cava and the presence of an associated thrombus [2] .

2. Patient demographics

1. Age

The average age of our patients, at the time of diagnosis of SCS of origin was 60.2 ± 11.3 years. In the literature, most authors report an average age ranging from 56.6 at 60.5 years (table I)

Table 49: Average age during SCS :

Author / study	Average age	Extremes
Kazdaghli BE (16)	56,7	[40-86]
D.Da Ines (6)	60,5	[44-81]
N.F lires (17)	56,6	[21-74]
L. Fekih (2)	57,8	[40-86]
Lynn D (7)	58	---
Richie CL chan (18)	65	[3-91]
Our series	60,2	[28-88]

This could be explained by the average age at onset of PBC, which according to data from the cancer register (North Tunisia) is 61.5 years [6,19]. According to studies, the median age at diagnosis of PBC is between 60 and 70 years [19,20, 21].

2. Type

The majority of studies of SCS of pulmonary neoplastic origin report frequently predominantly male (table II).

Table 50: Gender distribution during the SCS :

Author / study	Men (%)
Kazdhagli BE (16)	100
N.F Pires (17)	83,3
Fekih L (22)	100
D.Da Ines (6)	61,7
Lynn D (7)	100
Our series	98,1

This male predominance is explained by the high frequency of occurrence of CBP in men [19,23].

3. Smoking

The main risk factor for PBC remains smoking, which explains the high frequency of patients who smoke in the various studies of DBS associated with a pulmonary malignancy [16,17]. Smoking intoxication is often significant, with a mean of over 40 PA in several studies [16,17]. In our series it was 55.1 BP.

3. Clinical characteristics

1. Medical history

1.1.COPD

There is a frequent association between COPD and PBC, due to the fact that these two diseases share the same risk factor (smoking). This association varies from study to study. In our series, 23.1% of our patients had COPD (Table III).

Table 51: History of COPD in patients with PBC

Authors	COPD (%)
Jindal (24)	20,2
Imperatory (25)	30
Our series	23,1

1.2.Tuberculosis lung

Pleuropulmonary sequelae of tuberculosis are a risk factor for lung cancer. This risk increases with the age of the lesions [26]. In our series, a history of pulmonary tuberculosis was found in 5 cases (4.6%).

1.3. Neoplasia

Among the risk factors for developing PBC, a family history of cancer is a determining factor. Genetic predisposition interferes with other risk factors in the development of PBC. In our series, 10 patients (9, 25%) had a family history of cancer. This rate varies between 4% and 16% according to studies [19, 27, 28].

2. Deadline for consultation

The mean time between the onset of symptoms consistent with PBC or DBS and the first consultation was 59.2 days. This period is often quite long, varying between 41 and 99 days [19, 29,30].

3. Clinical manifestations linked to SCS

In the state phase, SCS has no etiological specificity, apart from the accompanying signs. The manifestations of SCS are triggered or aggravated by all circumstances that increase pressure in the superior vena cava (SVC), namely anteflexion, decubitus, and exertion, particularly of the upper limbs. Asymptomatic forms in which SCS is diagnosed on imaging are rare according to the literature [2, 31, 32]. In our series, obstruction of the SVC was symptomatic in 58.3% of cases and radiological findings in 41.7% of cases. DBS was indicative of PBC in 45 patients, which is consistent with the literature (Table IV).

Table 52: Frequency of revelatory SCS in PBC

Study	Frequency of revealing SCS (%)
D.Da Ines [6]	52.9
L.Fekih [22]	60
Our series	41.7

SCS was metachronous in 18 patients with a mean time to onset of 30 days. Malignant SCS progresses rapidly, with an average of 2 to 3 weeks between onset and detection [17, 22, 33,34].

3.1. Clinical signs

SCS is a group of signs and symptoms secondary to obstruction of SCV drainage and increased venous pressure in upstream territories. These signs are varied and inconsistent and can be grouped into 3 categories: respiratory, haemodynamic and neurological.

3.1.1. Signs respiratory

Dyspnoea, of variable intensity, is due either to airway oedema, oedema and stasis in the respiratory centres, or to the PBC itself. In our series, dyspnoea was found in 47 patients (43.5% of cases).The cough was often of irritant origin. It was reported by 56 patients (51.8%), which is in line with the data in the literature (38-70%). Chest pain and haemoptysis are most often due to PBC. Dysphonia and stridor may be due to venous stasis.

3.1.2. Neurological signs :

Neurological symptoms, linked to venous stasis in the nerve centres, include headaches, dizziness, tinnitus, drowsiness, obnubilation, syncope and even coma.

3.1.3. Signs haemodynamics

These physical signs are often suggestive of SCS.

•**Oedema:** the most constant and earliest sign. Initially, it is a simple filling of the supra-clavicular hollows, an increase in the volume of the neck and swelling of the eyelids. Then the oedema progressively increases, creating the classic "pilgrim's cape" appearance and infiltrating the whole of the upper neck and face, the upper limbs and the upper chest. In the face, the oedema affects the eyelids, cheeks, parotid region and tongue, which becomes thick, forcing the patient to keep his mouth open. The facial oedema found in 68.2% of our patients is consistent with the data in the literature (Table V) [2, 7, 17, 32].

Table 53: Clinical signs in SCS

Fréquence (%)	Intervalle (%)	
Hémodynamiques		
- Œdème des membres supérieur	82	60-100
- Turgescence des veines jugulaires	46	14-75
- Turgescence des veines jugulaires	63	27-86
- Circulation veineuse collatérale	53	39-67
- Pléthore facial	20	13-23
- Signes oculaires	2	0-3
Respiratoires		
- Dyspnée	54	23-74
- Toux	54	38-70
- Dysphonie	17	15-20
- Stridor	4	0-5
Neurologiques		
- Syncope	10	8-13
- Céphalées	9	6-11
- Vertiges	6	2-10
- Confusion	4	0-5
- Obnubilation	2	0-3

•**Turgidity of the jugular veins:** This turgidity can be seen at rest or when coughing. It has been found in 27 to 92% of patients, depending on the series, and in 38% of cases.

•**Cyanosis:** located in the cervico-facial region (lips, cheekbones, earlobes), is generally frustrating at the beginning and becomes general at an advanced stage. It was noted in 7.9% of our patients, a result close to that reported in the literature (13-45%).

•**Collateral venous circulation:** defined by the appearance ofa superficial thoraco-abdominal or peri-scapular collateral venous network. The frequency of this haemodynamic sign varies between 38% and 67% according to different studies.

3.2.Signs of severity

The clinical picture may be discrete or life-threatening, particularly in cases of laryngeal oedema (stridor, inspiratory dyspnoea) or cerebral oedema (drowsiness, coma, confusion) [2]. The severity of the superior vena cava syndrome is related to the degree of obstruction of the SVC and the the speed at which it sets in [35, 36, 37]. In our study, eight patients (12.7% of cases) presented signs of respiratory and haemodynamic severity such as inspiratory dyspnoea, significant desaturation, signs of struggle and cyanosis.

4. Anatomopathological data

1. Diagnostic confirmation :

Bronchial fibroscopy offers a direct approach to the diagnosis of endoscopically visible lung cancers. According to the literature, the histological type can be determined by bronchial biopsy, bronchial lavage or brushing in 48 to 80% of cases. % of cases [7,38]. Imaging-guided trans-thoracic biopsy is the second method of histological confirmation for peripheral lung tumours, with a sensitivity of 72% to 99% and a specificity of 91% to 100% [7,38]. It was performed in 17.5% of our patients, a result close to that described in the literature (22.2 to 30%) [19, 39, 40].

2. Anatomopathology

According to various studies, small cell lung carcinoma (SCLC) accounts for one-third of the pulmonary neoplastic causes of SCS, with variations ranging from 12% to 43% [7, 41, 42, 43, 44, 45].In fact, it is the histological type that most frequently causes SCS. In our series, CPC accounted for 40.7% of SCS (Table VI).

Table 54: Histological distribution of bronchial cancers in the SCS

Authors	Lyn D(7)	Fekih L(22)	D. Dalnes(6)	N. Piers(17)	Our series
NSCLC	50 %	55 %	79 %	45%	X %
C. Epidermoid	---	5 %	48 %	28,3%	29,9 %
ADK	---	15 %	37 %	16,7%	
Large cell carcinoma	---	35 %	14,8 %		
cells					
CPC	22 %	30 %	15%	41,7%	40,7%

According to Bellfkih et al [2], 10% of patients with CPC will develop SCS compared with only 2% with NSCLC. This is often disseminated CPC (61% of cases) [46,47]. In our series, CPC was diffuse in 28.7% of our patients. NSCLC account for 43-79% of malignant etiologies of SCS [6,7,22]. In our study, 64 patients had NSCLC: 29.6% squamous cell carcinoma and 25.9% adenocarcinoma. In our series, all patients with NSCLC were locally advanced or metastatic, with TNM stage IV in 32.4% of cases.

5. Imaging and exploration of the SCS

SCS is diagnosed clinically, while imaging is used to determine the characteristics of the stenosis, to provide information about the aetiology and thus to guide treatment. However, in some cases, it can provide an early diagnosis of DBS when the obstruction is still asymptomatic or when clinical signs are frustrated. Furthermore, in PBC, imaging is part of the extension work-up and enables the monitoring of neoplasia [43, 47,48].

1. Chest X-ray

Chest radiography was performed in all our patients. It is of limited value in the positive diagnosis of SCS, as it sometimes shows signs suggestive of SCS (dilatation of the aortic nipple [49,50], dilatation of the left brachiocephalic venous trunk or the azygos and costal erosions). With regard to aetiological diagnosis, chest X-rays are still very useful, showing abnormalities in 84% of cases [13]. In our series, 85.2% of patients presented with hilar opacities (33.3%), mediastino-pulmonary opacities (25%) or right intra-parenchymal opacities (20.4%). Mediastinal enlargement was found in 12% of cases.

2. Thoracic computed tomography (CT)

Chest CT with contrast injection remains the key examination in cases of suspected SCS [51], with sensitivity and specificity close to 100% [52,53].
This examination makes it possible to diagnose upper venous obstructions at a sub-clinical stage and thus initiate early treatment and improve prognosis. In our series, 45 patients were asymptomatic. It provides an objective view of the characteristics of the stenosis of the superior vena cava (location, length, degree, relationship with the right atrium, associated presence of an endoluminal thrombus, analysis of the collateral circulation, etc.) and provides a basis for orienting the aetiology by visualising an invasive mediastino-hilar process and locoregional and distant extension [2, 22, 54]. The thoracic scanner is also used for therapeutic monitoring of obstruction and bronchial cancer [43,48].

3. Magnetic resonance imaging

MRI is also an effective technique for diagnosing the causative lesion, and can be used to differentiate between a tumour with vascular invasion (thrombus, etc.) and a tumour with vascular invasion (thrombus, etc.). tumour) of a tumour causing venous compression with thrombosis at the site of the tumour. contact but without invading the vein wall [22]. However, the role of MRI remains limited due to the poor tolerance of decubitus and the frequent presence of dyspnoea. It is not currently indicated unless there is a contraindication to phleboscan [2,15].

4. Ultrasound and Doppler venous

These are non-invasive imaging techniques that are rarely used in the exploration of Upper cellar obstructions. Doppler ultrasound does not provide an optimal study of the SVC due to the chondrosternal bone and gas interface. It is indicated in cases of suspected thrombus [15]. Ultrasound and Doppler exploration is therefore limited to that of the supraclavicular and jugular veins in search of any indirect signs of venous obstruction. Superior vena cava phlebography, which was long considered to be the reference examination for assessing SCS, has now been superseded by phleboscanning. It remains useful during endovascular procedures for the placement of an endovascular prosthesis or in the event of in situ thrombolysis [2].

6. Treatment

The therapeutic management of tumour-induced SCS must be multidisciplinary and will depend on the severity of symptoms, the type of tumour and the patient's prognosis. The aims of treatment are to reduce symptoms and improve patient survival.

1. Treatment symptomatic

Symptomatic measures must be systematic. They help to improve the clinical signs and enable a check-up to be carried out in good conditions in patients in a precarious condition.These measures include resting in a seated or semi-seated position with the head elevated in order to reduce hydrostatic pressure, thereby reducing oedema and promoting venous drainage [14, 22]. However, there are no data confirming that The effectiveness of this manoeuvre is questionable, but it is simple and risk-free. What's more, it reduces dyspnoea by lowering the pressure in the SCV. Fluid restriction also helps to reduce oedema [2,7]. Oxygen therapy was indicated in hypoxic patients: 13.4% in our series. Symptomatic treatment involved medication (corticosteroids, anticoagulants and diuretics) and decompressive thoracic radiotherapy in 38.8% of our patients.

1.1.Treatment

1.1.1. The corticosteroid therapy

Corticosteroid therapy is often prescribed in cases of SVC obstruction for its anti-oedematous and anti-inflammatory properties. It is used as a first-line treatment while awaiting the results of imaging and histology. Corticosteroid therapy also helps to reduce oedema induced by radiotherapy [2, 55, 56]. However, a review of the literature does not classify corticosteroid therapy as an effective treatment on its own in the management of SCS [14, 17, 22, 56, 57, 58]. In our series, corticosteroid therapy was present in all our patients from the onset of SCS.

1.1.2. Treatment anticoagulant

Thromboembolic events are frequent in SCS, reaching up to 38%, so anticoagulation could help reduce their incidence, while heparin, mainly low molecular weight, could have anti-tumour properties [2, 59]. In vitro, it has been shown to inhibit angiogenesis and interfere with the metastatic process, a benefit that has also been observed in several studies [59,60]. However, there are currently no data demonstrating the benefits of prophylactic anticoagulation in the presence of SCS. In the absence of thrombus visualised on imaging, the use

of anticoagulant treatment is controversial due to the following factors However, it is often prescribed to avoid associated thrombosis of the SVC and to maintain the freedom of the collateral network [42,61]. Factors predictive of the efficacy of anticoagulant treatment in cases of constituted cruciate thrombosis are recent thrombosis and thrombosis associated with an implantable chamber [2].
The different molecules used are unfractionated heparin, low molecular weight heparin and heparin for the treatment of acute myocardial infarction. anti-Vit K in certain cases. In our series, anticoagulant treatment was prescribed in only 30 patients (27.7%).

1.1.3. The diuretics

Diuretics are sometimes prescribed for their anti-oedematous properties in the treatment of SCS, whatever the aetiology. However, their efficacy remains poorly demonstrated in the literature [14, 17, 22, 32,62]. Only one patient in our series was treated with diuretics.

1.2. thrombolysis

Thrombolysis is recommended if the SCS is linked to a crucial occlusive thrombosis of the SVC.

If there are no contraindications, streptokinase, urokinase and tissue plasminogen activator are recommended. These are exogenous plasminogen activators that produce fibrinolysis by activating the body's natural fibrinolytic system. After thrombolysis, preventive anticoagulant treatment with heparin may be prescribed. According to the literature, the efficacy of thrombolysis varies from 22% to 100% [35, 63, 64, 65]. It varies according to the type of fibrinolytic product used and the age of the clot; the more recent the thrombus, the more effective it is [64].
In addition, thrombolysis is more effective in the case of a central venous catheter, because thrombolysis can be delivered directly to the clot via the implantable chamber catheter. Thrombolysis therefore appears to be an effective treatment for recent cruciate thrombosis of the SVC, but it is associated with high morbidity and mortality. Indications for SCS of pulmonary neoplastic origin are rare. In our series, no patient underwent thrombolysis. Tumour invasion and extrinsic compression by the tumour are often associated. In these cases, thrombolysis does not appear to be the treatment of choice.

1.3.Treatment endovascular

First described in 1986, percutaneous placement of an endovascular prosthesis in the superior vena cava position restores continuity of the SVC, removes the obstacle to SVC return and removes the obstacle to brachiocephalic venous return [2].This is a rapid, minimally invasive procedure, often preceded by angioplasty, but not always. The response rate after endovascular stent grafting is 90-100%, with the advantage of rapid relief of symptoms such as headache, cyanosis and oedema [2,45, 66,65], with a response rate of 75-100% [7].
Its efficacy is independent of histology [2,67]. However, if the obstruction of the SVC is due to extrinsic compression, the efficacy is better than if it is due to tumour thrombosis [68].In the event of thrombus, thrombolysis can be performed during an endovascular procedure using in situ injection. The thrombus can also be fragmented using a guide. Unfortunately, the high cost of endovascular prosthesis means that it is not widely used.

1.4.Radiotherapy

As the majority of bronchopulmonary tumours that cause SCS are radiosensitive, radiotherapy was long considered to be the primary treatment for SCS. It reduces the signs of venous obstruction by reducing the volume of the tumour mass [2,16].A systemic review of the literature has demonstrated the role of radiotherapy in achieving a clinical response in 78% of patients with lung cancer and 63% of patients treated for NSCLC after 3 to 15 days of irradiation [2, 7, 14, 45]. Improvement is sometimes visible as early as the first 72 hours [7, 8, 69, 70].Some authors have recommended emergency radiotherapy for severe SCS with signs of severity, even in the absence of a histological diagnosis [7, 16, 17]. This could make anatomopathological analysis more difficult with pot-radiotherapy. In the study by Loffler et al, histological diagnosis by biopsy after initial irradiation of SCS was established in only 58% of patients [71]. At present, it is accepted that radiotherapy is not a therapeutic emergency in cases of SCS [7, 22, 72, 73,74]. The choice of dose and volume to be irradiated will depend on the aim of the treatment (curative or palliative) and the type of histology. In patients for whom a curative strategy is being considered, doses of 36 to 70 Gray are recommended (depending on the histological type), often with conventional fractionation (1.8 to 2 Gray per fraction) in order to limit late toxicity. In the case of palliative radiotherapy, the choice of dose and fractionation will depend essentially on the patient's prognosis and general condition. Hypofractionated radiotherapy is then indicated, and the different regimens found in the literature appear to be equivalent in terms of clinical benefit [45,75].Decompressive radiotherapy uses fractions at higher doses than those used in conventional radiotherapy and for a shorter duration. This can lead to greater toxicity [75,76]. However, thanks to the widespread use of conformal radiotherapy and recent advances in radiotherapy, in particular stereotaxy and image guidance, optimal protection of organs at risk and better coverage of the target volume can be achieved [77,78]. Decompressive radiotherapy is proving to be an effective treatment for SCS associated with bronchopulmonary cancers. The success rate varies from 64% to 80% depending on the series [2, 4, 22, 34, 35]. The response is complete in 15 to 23% of cases and incomplete in half [7, 79, 80, 81, 82]. In our series, 66% of our patients who received thoracic decompressive radiotherapy improved their SCS symptoms, with a complete response in 25% of cases and a partial response in 75%, results comparable to those in the literature [7,16]. Side effects of radiotherapy include initial aggravation by radio-induced oedema, dysphagia, nausea, chest burns and radiodermatitis, post-radiation fibrosis and bone marrow toxicity. The higher the fractions, the more frequent the complications [80]. In our series, 18 patients (26%) developed side effects following radiotherapy. Recurrence of SCS was noted in two patients following tumour progression. These recurrences were resistant to further radiotherapy [83,84].

2. The chemotherapy

Chemotherapy is the treatment of choice for SCS secondary to pulmonary neoplasia. In this case, it is essential to establish a histological diagnosis before starting chemotherapy. The efficacy of treatment varies according to the histology of the bronchopulmonary cancer. According to a review of the literature, chemotherapy leads to a clinical response with complete improvement in DBS symptoms in approximately 80% of lung cancer patients and 40% of NSCLC patients [7, 22, 45]. In fact, in the study by Roswell et al[45] of patients with inaugural DBS, chemotherapy improved symptoms in 77% of patients with CBPC, with only 17% relapsing. The time to clinical response was identical to that for radiotherapy and ranged from 7 to 15 days [45].

In our series, the clinical response to chemotherapy was noted in 60% of patients with CBPC and 26% of those with CBNPC, results comparable to those in the literature.Recurrence of SCS without chemotherapy was noted in 6% of our patients. This recurrence is due to tumour progression. Combining chemotherapy with radiotherapy, in the case of localised NSCLC or small tumours, reduces the relapse rate. For NSCLC, the indications for chemotherapy alone or in combination with radiotherapy depend on the stage of the tumour. Chemo-radiotherapy for stage III B and chemotherapy for stage IV, in which case radiotherapy is only indicated for palliative purposes to reduce obstruction of the SVC. A review of two randomised studies and 44 observational studies showed that there was no clinically significant difference in the degree of improvement in DBS between chemotherapy alone, radiotherapy and combined chemo-radiotherapy [7, 45, 85]. There is a significant risk of complications associated with chemotherapy. These are essentially haematological, digestive, renal and skin toxicity [2,16] and, because of the hyperhydration associated with it, chemotherapy can increase venous engorgement and thus increase the symptoms of SVC obstruction [2,46]. In our series, Carboplatin was used in 5 of our patients to avoid this undesirable effect. In the literature, as in our series, the side effects associated with chemotherapy are significant [16, 46, 54, 86] in frail patients with a short life expectancy.

3. The surgery

In a palliative situation, surgery can remove obstruction of the SVC by performing a bypass between the internal jugular vein and the right auricle, most frequently, or between the internal jugular (or axillary) vein and the femoral vein to provide extra-anatomical vascularisation using a polytetrafluoroethylene prosthesis [7,87]. This technique has now been superseded by endo-vascular treatment and may be reserved for patients who have failed the latter. Curative surgical treatment consists of a pneumonectomy extended to the SVC with lymph node dissection.Surgery for obstructions of the SVC uses a wide sternotomy approach with or without transverse cervicotomy or posterolateral thoracotomy. The surgical procedure consists of either :

- Disobstruction with or without angioplasty of the superior vena cava.
- Resection and replacement of the blocked portion of the vein.
- A bypass without removal of the obstructed vein.

This treatment of SVC obstruction may or may not be associated with resection of the bronchopulmonary tumour.

Surgery for obstruction of the SVC is associated with significant morbidity and mortality [16, 42, 72, 88] and intraoperative mortality is estimated at between 6.5 and 30% [67]. The good results of surgical treatment were found for minor obstructions of the SVC, NSCLC and patients in good general condition. There was no indication for surgery in our series.

7. Survival and prognostic factors

1. Survival overall

Despite advances in treatment and rapid management of tumour-induced SCS bronchopulmonary, this entity continues to have a poor prognosis. The median survival varies according to the authors from 6 to 9 months, results which are consistent with our study where the median survival is 7 months. The 2-year survival rate in our series was 6% (Table VII).

Table 55: Overall survival

Authors	Median of survival (months)	Survival to 1 year in (%)	2 years in (%)	5 years in (%)
S. Bellefqih [7]	6 - 9	---	5	2
N. F. Pives [17]	8	---	---	---
R. CL Chan [18]	6,5	---	---	---
F. L. Ampil [89]	8	36	7	2
S Mose [90]	9,5	[17 - 35]	---	---
F. A. Bristgens [91]	7,8	---	---	---
Our series	7	22	6	---

According to the literature, life expectancy for patients with neoplastic SCS is 6 months, but this estimate varies widely depending on the underlying neoplastic conditions [7, 90,92]. According to some authors, SCS in itself is not a poor prognostic factor, since overall survival does not differ for PBC of the same histological type and stage according to the presence or absence of SCS [7, 17, 18].In fact, SCS rarely causes death, which is most often secondary to tumour progression. Moreover, if laryngeal oedema does occur, it is often difficult to distinguish between death secondary to the laryngeal oedema itself or to tracheal compression, which is very frequently associated. Similarly, in the rare cases reported of death following cerebral oedema, the presence of associated metastases is generally poorly documented, although the incidence of metastases may be particularly high in the case of SCS [2].

2. Prognostic factors

2.1.Study univariate

2.1.1. Age

The majority of studies have found that age is an important factor influencing the prognosis of SCS of pulmonary neoplastic origin, with survival deteriorating with age [2, 44, 62, 73]. In a study of 104 patients with tumour-induced SCS, RCL chan demonstrated that an age of 50 years or less was significantly associated with longer survival in a univariate study with p = 0.000 [18].However, in our series, age 60 or less was correlated with a shorter median survival (6 months versus 7 months) but the difference was statistically insignificant. This could be explained by the predominance of the 61-70 age group. According to S. Mose et al. Mose et al [100], age is not a prognostic factor.

2.1.2. Gender

In our series, no significant difference in survival was found according to sex. The predominance of males in our population may explain these results.There are no studies in the literature that have investigated the prognostic value of gender in lung neoplastic SCS.

2.1.3. Smoking

Smoking is the main risk factor for bronchopulmonary cancer. Several studies have shown that the survival of non-smoking patients with SCS of pulmonary tumour origin is better than that of smokers. Indeed, N.F. Piers et al found a better overall survival in non-smokers with a significant difference (p = 0.038) [17]. Similarly, in the study of 104 patients with malignant obstruction of the SVC, survival was significantly longer in non-smokers: 35.7 months versus 3.4 months in smokers (p = 0.012). This was partly explained by the comorbidities associated with smoking and resistance to treatment, particularly chemotherapy. In our series, the absence of smoking was correlated with better survival in non-smokers, but the difference was statistically insignificant.

2.1.4. Weight loss

The presence of recent weight loss in our patients did not influence median survival, which was comparable to the median survival of patients without weight loss (7 months in both groups), but the difference was not significant. There are no studies implicating weight loss as a prognostic factor in DBS of pulmonary neoplastic origin.

2.1.5. Condition

Assessing the patient's general condition is an essential step in the management of lung cancer with SCS. The treatment decision depends on the patient's general condition.The use of less aggressive therapeutic means is recommended when the PS is greater than or equal to 2. Several studies have shown that good general health is associated with better survival [2, 17, 24, 62, 73, 93, 100]. Indeed, according to N. F. Piers et al, a good PS of 0 or 1 was positively correlated with overall survival with a statistically significant difference (p = 0, 033) [7]. In our series, patients with a PS of two or more had a shorter survival than patients in good general condition (p<0.001).

Table 56: Survival according to WHO PS score

Authors	Survival by PS score	P
F. L Ampil [89]	NS	p = 0,12
S. Mose [100]	S	p < 0,004
NF Piers [17]	S	p = 0,033
Our series	S	p < 0,001

2.1.6. Respiratory function

According to a review of the literature, the degree of bronchial obstruction has a negative influence on survival in patients with PBC associated with chronic obstructive pulmonary disease. This association is frequent given that the two diseases share the same risk factor (smoking) [94,95]. However, the various studies of SCS of pulmonary neoplastic origin have not mentioned respiratory function (bronchial obstruction and chronic hypoxaemia) as a prognostic factor. In our patients, a FEV1 $\geq$ 70% was associated with a better survival with a difference statically significant (p = 0.04). In addition, median survival was shorter (4 $\pm$ 0.5 months versus 8 $\pm$ 0.7 months) in cases of chronic respiratory failure (p = 0.01).

2.1.7. Type histological

A review of the literature on survival according to histological type showed variable results (table VIII) Several studies have shown that the survival of patients with NSCLC is better than that of patients with HNSCC [17,91].
PBC was correlated with better survival. In our series, patients with PBC had a

longer median survival than those with NSCLC (8.5 months versus 5 months) with a statistically significant difference.

Table 57: Survival by histological type

Auteurs	Survie CPC vs CNPC
N. F Piers [17]	S
D. Lynn [7]	S
A. Felix [91]	S
FL. Ampil [89]	NS
Notre série	S

S : significatif

NS : non significatif

2.1.8. Assessment of extension

Regardless of the histological type of tumour, the presence of metastasis is an important prognostic factor for SCS of neoplastic origin [2, 17, 62, 73, 93]. According to N. F Piers, the absence of metastasis is positively correlated with overall patient survival with a statistically significant difference (p = 0, 027) [17].Survival in our patients was better for localised or locally advanced stages, but the difference was statistically insignificant. However, the number of metastatic sites of two or more was significantly associated with shorter survival compared with patients with a single metastasis (5 months versus 8 months) (p = 0.01). There are no studies on the prognostic importance of the number of metastatic sites in SCS of pulmonary malignant origin. This factor essentially reflects the proliferative and aggressive capacity of the underlying tumour.

2.1.9. Superior venous syndrome symptomatic

According to several authors, SCS in itself is not a poor prognostic factor. In fact, overall survival in bronchopulmonary cancer of the same histological type and stage is identical and does not differ according to the presence or absence of signs of DBS [7, 17, 18].Contrary to Martin SJ [96] who found in his study that SCS was a poor prognostic factor with an overall survival of 5 months. Similarly, F. L. Ampil [89] reported that DBS was a poor predictive factor. In our study, the median survival in symptomatic DBS was 5.5 months compared with 8 months in the absence of symptoms, but the difference was statistically insignificant. Severity of DBS was a poor prognostic factor with significantly reduced survival.

2.1.10. Treatment of bronchopulmonary cancer

Specific anti-cancer treatment is a parameter of definite prognostic value. Chemotherapy provides symptom control, improves quality of life and prolongs survival [97, 98, 99].According to Lynn D [7], a complete regression of SVC obstruction symptoms can be seen under systematic chemotherapy in 80% of patients with CBPC and 40% of those with CBNPC. However, Rowell NP, in his systemic review of 2 randomised studies and 44 observational studies, concluded that in patients with bronchopulmonary cancer, there was no significant difference in DBS remission rate and overall survival according to the treatment prescribed: chemotherapy alone or chemo-radiotherapy [45]. In our study, a better survival was noted with chemotherapy (8 months) with a statistically significant difference in the case of NSCLC ($p = 0.003$) and in the case of SCLC ($p < 0.001$).

2.1.11. Treatment of SCS

2.1.11.1. Decompressive radiotherapy

For a long time, malignant SCS was considered an extreme medical emergency requiring urgent decompressive radiotherapy to reduce the size of the bronchopulmonary tumour and thus reduce obstruction of the SVC. This reduces the symptoms of SCS in 90% of cases [91].S. Mose in his retrospective study of SCS in irradiated cancer patients showed that the group of patients who received complete decompressive radiotherapy had better survival than those who stopped treatment because of toxicity, with a median overall survival of 5 months versus 2.7 months [100].Furthermore, according to Z. Wang, survival was better in SCS patients with lung cancer who received low-dose radiotherapy (18.7 months) than in patients who received high-dose radiotherapy (15 months). However, according to N.F. Piers [17], emergency decompressive irradiation even before anatomopathological proof can make histological diagnosis by biopsy difficult at a later date [17]. In our series, decompressive thoracic radiotherapy was performed in 37 of our patients with a median survival of 6 months, but the correlation was statistically insignificant.

2.1.11.2. Medical treatment for SCS

Corticosteroid treatment is frequently prescribed for SCS of neoplastic origin, although its therapeutic effect has not been well studied in the literature. Its beneficial role in reducing oedema and obstruction of the SVC remains unclear.
In an observational study including 107 patients with SCS, clinical improvement was comparable between patients treated with corticosteroids and diuretics and

those who received neither treatment [62].In our patients, the prognostic impact of symptomatic medical treatment was not not statistically significant. The main independent prognostic factors vary from study to study.The study by N. F. Piers identified independent factors for a good prognosis: good general condition (PS = 0 or 1), absence of tumour metastases and absence of smoking [17]. In fact, the performance index is an important prognostic factor found in multivariate analysis in several studies [2,17, 93].Smoking was a risk factor for mortality [17, 18]. Tumour stage and absence of metastasis were factors positively correlated with overall survival. In our series, the predictive factors for DBS mortality in bronchopulmonary cancer were: male sex, smoking, deterioration in general condition, the presence of two or more metastases and the presence of signs of DBS severity.

CHAPTER 5
CONCLUSION

The superior vena cava syndrome is a group of clinical manifestations linked to the interruption of the superior vena cava current in relation to vessel compression, invasion or thrombosis. There are many aetiologies, but they are dominated by neoplastic causes, mainly of bronchopulmonary origin. The aim of this retrospective study was to establish the clinical, radiological and evolutionary profile, as well as the therapeutic management of PBC-related SCS, whatever the histological type, to assess survival, and to identify and analyse the various prognostic factors. One hundred and eight patients with SCS complicating primary bronchial cancer were hospitalised in the Pneumology Department at Fattouma Bourguiba between 1990 and 2015. The results obtained from this study show: There was a clear male predominance (98.1%), the average age was At 60.2 years of age, smoking was found in 68.5% of cases, with an average consumption of 55.1 PA. Superior cava syndrome was indicative of the neoplasm in 41.7% of cases. It was metachronous in 16.6% of cases. Clinically, the symptoms were dominated by facial oedema, filling of the supra-clavicular hollows, collateral venous circulation and turgidity of the jugular veins.Signs of severity such as cerebral or laryngeal oedema did not complicate the SCS, but signs of respiratory severity, in particular dyspnoea, accompanied 6 patients. Chest X-rays were used to orientate the diagnosis, and essentially showed hilar or mediastino-pulmonary opacity in 33.3% and 25% of cases respectively.Bronchial fibroscopy is used to visualise the tumour and take histopathological samples. It revealed a pathological appearance in 90.4% of cases. The lesions were mainly located on the right, and the right upper lobar bronchus was the most affected (67%). The most common histological type of SCS was CPC (40.7%).Thoracic CT with PDC is the key examination in cases of SCS, enabling a topographical diagnosis to be made, locoregional extension to be determined, treatment to be planned and post-treatment monitoring to be carried out. The most common scan finding was tumour invasion of the SCV (62.2%). MRI is considered to be an alternative means of diagnosing SCS, but its use is limited by the poor tolerance of decubitus and the frequent presence of dyspnoea. It is indicated mainly in cases where CT is contraindicated. Doppler ultrasonography is not widely used in the investigation of superior venous obstructions. Superior vena cava phlebography, long considered to be the key examination, is now associated with CT and is indicated during endovascular procedures or in the event of discrepancies between clinical findings and imaging techniques (CT, MRI).The treatment of SCS is multidisciplinary, involving drug therapy, the efficacy of which is still uncertain, radiotherapy, which is considered the gold standard for the treatment of SCS as it is highly radiosensitive, chemotherapy and endovascular treatment, which is playing an increasingly important role. Its role is essentially symptomatic, with rapid improvement in symptoms, and its combination with chemotherapy and radiotherapy will help to control the disease and reduce recurrence. Short-term prognosis depends on the consequences of cerebral and laryngeal oedema and the existence of complications (tracheal compression, pleuropericardial effusion). Long-term prognosis depends on the underlying aetiology, which in our study was PBC.

REFERENCES BIBLIOGRAPHIQUES

1. Limal N, Wechsler B. Superior cava syndromes. Sang Thrombose Vaisseaux 2006; 18, n° 1: 17-22.
2. Bellefqih S, Khalil J, Mezouri I, Afif M, Elmajjaoui S, Kebdani T, Benjaafar N. Superior cava syndrome of malignant origin. Revue de Pneumologie Clinique (2014) 70, 343-352.
3. Hunter W. The history of an aneurysm of the aorta with some remarks on aneurysm in general. Med Obs Soc Phys Lond 1757; 323.
4. Davenport D, Ferree C, Blake D, Raben M. Radiation therapy in treatment of superior vena cava obstruction. Cancer 1978; 42: 2600-03.
5. Parish JM, Marshke RF Jr, Dines DE, Lee RE.Etiologic considerations in superior vena cava syndrome. Mayo Clin Proc 1985 ; 56 :407-413.
6. Ines Da D, Chabrot P, Cassagnes L, Merle P, Filaire M, Ravel A, Garcier JM, Boyer

L. Endovascular treatment of neoplastic superior vena cava syndrome: a case report of 34 patients. J Radiol 2008; 89:881-90.
7. Wilson LD, Detterbeck FC, Yahalom J. Superior vena cava syndrome with malignant causes.N Engl J Med 2007 ;356 :1862-9.
8. Armstrong BA, Perez CA, Simpson JR, Hederman MA. Role of irradiation in the management of superior vena cava syndrome.Int J Radiat Oncol Biol Phys 1987; 13:531- 9.
9. Chen JC, Bongard F, Klein SR. A contemporary perspective on superior vena cava syndrome. Am J Surg 1990; 160:207-11.
10. Rice TW, Rodriguez RM, Light RW. The superior vena cava syndrome: clinical characteristics and evolving etiology.Medicine (Baltimore) 2006; 85:37.
11. Lepper PM, Ott SR,Hoppe H, Schumann C, stammberger U, Bugalho A, Frese S, Schmucking M, Blumstein NM, Diehm N, Bals R, Hamacher J. Superior vena cava syndrome in Thoracic malignancies. Respi Care 2011; 56(5):653-666.
12. Doty DB, Doty JR, and Jones KW. Bypass of superior vena cava: Fifteen years' experience with spiral vein grafts for obstruction of superior vena cava caused by benign disease. J Thorac Cardiovasc Surg 1990; 99:889-96.
13. Parish JM, Marsche RF Jr, Dines DE, Lee RE. Etiologic considerations in superior vena cava syndrome. Mayo Clin Proc 1981; 56:407-13.
14. Lacout A, Marcy P,Thariat J, Lacombe P, El hajjam M . Radio-anatomy of the superior vena cava syndrome and therapeutic orientations. Diagnostic and

interventional imaging (2012) 93; 569-577.
15. El hajjam, Lagrange C, Desperramons J, Hardit C, Binsse S, Lacombe P. Diagnostic and therapeutic imaging of the superior vena cava. EMC Radiologie et imagerie médicale -cardiovasculaire-thoracique -cervicale 2010; 32-225-F-20.
16. Kazdaghi Boukhris E. Superior cave syndrome and bronchopulmonary cancer: about 20 cases. Th D Med, Tunis 2009.
17. Pires NF, Morais A, Queiroga H.Superior vena cava syndrome as tumour presentation. Rev Port Pneumol 2010; 16 (1):73-88.
18. Chan RCL, Chan YC and Cheng SWK. Mid-and long term follow up experience in patients with malignant superior vena cava obstruction. Interactive cardiovascular and thoracic surgery 16 (2013) 455-458.
19. Blel S. Non-small cell lung cancer: survival and prognostic factors. ThD Med, Monastir 2015.
20. Blanchon F, Grivaux M, Collon T, Zureik M, Barbieux H, Bénichou-Flurin M et al. Epidemiology and management of primary bronchial cancer in French general hospitals, Rev Mak Respir 2002; 19(6)727-34.
21. Davidoff AJ, Tang M, Seal B, Edelman MJ. Chemotherapy and survival benefit in elderly patients with advanced non-small lung cancer. J Clin Oncol 2010; 28(13):2191- 7.
22. Fekih L, Boussouffara L, Fenniche S, Kasdaghli E, Belhabib D, Abdelghaffar H, Hassene H, Ben Miled K, Mezni F, Megdiche ML. La tunisie médicale 2010;Vol88(n°10).
23. Parkin DM, Bray F, Ferlay J, Pisani P. Global cancer statistics, 2002. CA. Cancer J Clin 2005;55(2):74-108.
24. Jindal SK, Behera D. Clinical spectrum of primary lung cancer. Review of Chandigarh experience of 10 years. Lung india 1990;8(2):94-8.
25. Imperatori A, Harrison RN, Leitch DN, Rovera F, Lepore G, Dionigi G, et al. Lung cancer in Teesside (UK) and Varese (Italy): a comparison of management and survival. Thorax 2006; 61(3):232-9.
26. Zheng W, Blot WJ, Liao ML, Wang ZX, Levin LI, Zhao JJ, et al. Lung cancer and prior tuberculosis infection in Shinghai.Br J.cancer 1987;56(4):501-6.
27. Nitadori J, Inoue M, Iwasaki M, Otani T, Sasazuki S, Nagai K, et al. Association between lung cancer incidence and family history of lung cancer: data from a large-scale population-based cohort study, the JPHC study. Chest 2006; 130(4):968-75.
28. Yang P, Allen MS, Aubry MC, Wampfler JA, Marks RS, Edell ES, et al. Clinical features of 5,628 primary lung cancer patients: experience at Mayo Clinic from 1997 to 2003.Chest 2005;128(1):452-62.

29. Smith SM, Campbell NC, Macleod U, Lee AJ, Raja A, Wyke S , et al. Factors contributing to the time taken to consult with symptoms of lung cancer: a cross-sectional study. Thorax 2009; 64(6):523-31.
30. Virally J, Choudat L, Chebbo M, Sartene R, Jagot J, Elhadadet A, et al. Epidemiology and management delays in 355 patients with bronchial cancer. Rev Mal Respir 2006;23(1 Pt 1):43-8.

31. Becthold RE, Wolfman NT, Karsteadt N et al. Superior vena cava obstruction :detection using CT- Radiology 1985; 157: 485-7.

32. Yu JB, Wilson LD, Detterbeck FC. Superior vena cava syndrome: a proposed classification system and algorithm for management. J Thorac Oncol 2008; 3:811-4.

33. Marlier S, Bonal J, Cellarier G, Bouchiat C, Talard PH, Dussarat GV. The Superior cava syndromes of benign aetiology. Presse Med 1996; 25: 12037.

34. Abner A. Approach to the patient who presents with superior vena cava obstruction. Chest 1993; 103: 394-97.
35. Jackson JE, Brooks DM. Stenting of superior vena cava obstruction. Clin. Radiol. 1994; 49: 202-8.
36. Hochrein J, Bashore TM, O'laughlin MP, Harrison JK. Percutaneous stenting of superior vena cava syndrome: case report and review of literature. Am. J. Med. 1998; 104: 78-84.

37. Kishi K, Sonomura T, Mitsuzane K, Nishida N, Yang RJ, Sato M, Yamada R, Shirai S, Kabayashi H. Self-expandable metallic stent therapy for superior vena cava syndrome: Clinical obstructions. Radiology 1993; 189: 531-35.
38. Mazzone P, Jain P, Arroliga AC, Matthay RA. Bronchoscopy and needle biopsy techniques for diagnosis and staging of lung cancer. Clin Chest Med 2002; 23(1) :137- 58.
39. Tlili F. Palliative chemotherapy of locally advanced and metastatic non-small cell lung carcinoma (series of 45 cases).ThD Med, Tunis;2010.
40. Ben Ali G. Treatment of primary non-microcellular bronchopulmonary cancer in locally advanced and metastatic stages: about 150 cases. ThD Med, Tunis; 2013.
41. Stock KW, Jacob AL, Proske M, Rochlitz C, and Steinbrich W. Treatment of malignant obstruction of the superior vena cava with self-expanding Wallstent. Thorax 1995; 50: 1151- 56.
42. Cheng S. Superior vena cava syndrome: a contemporary review of a historic disease. Cardiol Rev. 2009 Jan-Feb; 17(1):16-23.
43. Abner A. Approach to the patient who presents with superior vena cava

obstruction. Chest 1993; 103: 394-97.
44. Armstrong BA, Perez CA, Simpson JR, et al. Role of irradiation in the management of superior vena cava syndrome. Int. J. Radiat. Oncol. Biol. Phys. 1987; 13: 531-39.
45. Rowell NP, Gleeson FV. Steroids, radiotherapy, chemotherapy and stents for superior vena cava obstruction in carcinoma of the bronchus: a systematic review. Clin Oncol (R Coll Radiol) 2002; 14:338-51.
46. Urban T, Lebeau B, Chastang C, Leclerc P, Botto MJ, Sauvaget J. Superior vena cava syndrome in small cell lung cancer Arch. Intern. Med. 1993; 153: 384-87.
47. BOF M. Apport des endoprothèses autoexpansives dans le traitement du syndrome cave supérieur. Thesis of Medicine, Nancy I, 1994.
48. Coulomb M, Moro D, Lerumeur Y, Ranchoup Y, Rosepittet L, Brambilla C, et al. Place des nouvelles techniques d'imagerie médicales (TDM et IRM) dans la stratégie diagnostique du syndrome de la veine cave supérieure. Rev Mal Respir 1991; 8: 45-57.
49. Ball JB, Proto AV. The variable appearance of the left superior intercostal vein. Radiology 1982; 144: 445-52. 35- 50.
50. Carter MM, Tarr RW, Mazzer MJ, Caroll FE. The "Aortic Nipple" as a sign of impending superior vena cava syndrome. Chest 1985; 87: 775-77.
51. Engel IA, Auh YH, Rubenstein WA, Sniderman K, Whalen JP, Kazan E. CT diagnosis of mediastinal and thoracic inlet venous obstruction. Am J Roentgenol 1983; 141:521-26.
52. Becthold RE, Wolfman NT, Karsteadt N, et al. Superior vena cava obstruction :detection using CT- Radiology 1985; 157: 485-7.
53. Gooding GAW, Hightower DR, Moore EH, Dillon WP, Lipton MJ. Obstruction of superior vena cava or subclavian veins: sonographic diagnosis. Radiology 1986; 159: 663-65.
54. Cosmidis I. Contribution of CT to the diagnosis of superior vena cava syndrome in adults (about 42 cases). Medical thesis, Nancy, 1995.
55. Cohen R, Mena D, Carbajal-Mendoza R, Matos N, Karki N. Superior vena cava syndrome: a medical emergency? Int J Angiol. 2008; 17:43-46
56. Sculier J, Evans W, Feld R, et al. Superior vena caval obstruction syndrome in small cell lung cancer. Cancer. 1986; 57:847-851
57. Kvale PA, Selecky PA, Prakash UB. American College of chest Physicians. Palliative care in lung cancer: ACCP evidence-based clinical practice guidelines (2nd edition).Chest 2007; 132(suppl.3):3685-403S.

58. Brzezniak C, Oronsky B, Carter CA, Thilagar B, Caroen S, Zeman K.Superior vena cava syndrome in a patient with small-cell lung cancer: a case report. Case Rep Onco 2017; 10:252-257.
59. Marchetii M,Vignoli A, Russo L, Balducci D, Pagnoncelli M, Barbui T, et al. Endothelial capillary tube formation and cell proliferation induced by tumor cells are affected by low molecular weight heparins and unfractionated heparin.Thromb Res 2008;121:637-45.
60. Mousa SA. Low-molecular-weight heparins in thrombosis and cancer: emerging links.Cardiovasc Drug Rev 2004; 22:121-34.
61. Wan JF, Bezjak A. Superior vena cava syndrome.Emerg Med Clin North Am 2009; 27:243-55.
62. Schraufnagel DE, Hill R, Leech JA, Pare JA.Superior vena cava obstruction: is it a medical emergency? Am J Med 1981; 70:1169-74.
63. Rantis P, Littooy F. Successful treatment of prolonged superior vena cava syndrome with thrombolytic therapy: a case report. J. Vasc; Surg. 1994; 20: 108-03.
64. Gray B, Olin J, Graor R, Young W, Bartholomew J, Ruschhaupt W. Safety and efficacy of thromboembolytic therapy for superior vena cava syndrome. Chest 1991; 99: 54-59.
65. Rachapalli V, Boucher LM. Superior vena cava syndrome: Role of the interventionalist.Canadian Association of Radiologists Journal 65(2014) 168-176.
66.Hamzik J, Chudej J, Dzian A, Sokol J, K Ubisz P. Endovascular stenting in malignant obstruction of superior vena cava. International Journal of Surgery Case Reports 13(2015) 84-87.
67. Bergeron P, Reggi M, Jausseran JM, Huet R, Ferdani M, Martelet JP, Longefait H, Courbier F. Our experience of superior vena cava surgery. ANN. CH:Chir.Thorac.Cardio-vasc.1985;39:485-91.
68. Hennequin L, Fade O, Fays J, Bic JF, Jaaffar S, Bertal A, Anthoine D, Bernardac P. Superior vena cava stent placement: results with wallstent endoprothesis. Radiology 1995;196 :353-61.
69. Anderson PR, Coia LR. Fractionation and outcomes with palliative radiation therapy. Semin Radiat Oncol 2000; 10:191-199.
70. Pereira JR, Martins SJ, Ikari FK, Nikaedo SM, Gampel O. Neoadjuvant chemotherapy vs radiotherapy alone for superior vena cava syndrome (SVCS) due to non-small cell lung cancer (NSCLC): preliminary results of randomized phase II trial. Eur J Cancer 1999; 35: Suppl 4:260-260.
71. Loeffler JS, et al. Emergency prebiopsy radiation for mediastinal masses: impact on subsequent pathologic diagnosis and outcome. J Clin Oncol 1986;

4:716.
72. Chen JC, Bongard F, Klein SR. A contemporary perspective on superior vena cava syndrome. Am. J. Surg. 1990; 160: 207-11.
73. Yellin A, Rosen A, Reichert N, Liebermen Y. Superior vena syndrome: the myth, the facts. Am. Rev. Respir. Dis 1990; 141: 1114-8.
74. Urban T, Lebeau B, Chastang C, Leclerc P, Botto MJ, Sauvaget J. Superior vena cava syndrome in small cell lung cancer Arch. Intern. Med. 1993; 153: 384-87.
75. Rodriguez G, Videtic GM, Sur R, Bezjak A, Bradley J, Hahn CA, et al. Palliative thoracic radiotherapy in lung cancer: an American Society for Radiation Oncology evidence based clinical practice guideline. Pract Radiat Oncol 2011; 1: 60-71.
76. Stanford W, Jolles H, Ell S, Chiu LC. Superior vena cava obstruction: a venographic classification. AJR Am J Roentgenol 1987; 148:259-62.
77. Grutters JP, Kessels AG, Pijls-Johannesma M, De Ruysscher D, Joore MA, Lambin P. Comparison of the effectiveness of radiotherapy with photons, protons and carbon- ions for non-small cell lung cancer: a meta-analysis. Radiother Oncol 2010; 95:32-40.
78. Liao ZX, Komaki RR, Thames Jr HD, Liu HH, Tucker SL, Mohan R, et al. Influence of technologic advances on outcomes in patients with unresectable, locally advanced non-small-cell lung cancer receiving concomitant chemoradiotherapy. Int J Radiat Oncol Biol Phys 2010; 76:775-81.
79. Gauden SJ. Superior vena cava syndrome induced by bronchogenic carcinoma: is this an oncological emergency? Australas. Radiol. 1993; 37: 363-66.
80. Nicholson AA, Ettles D, Arnold A, Greenstone M, Dyet JF. Treatment of malignant superior vena cava obstruction: metal stents or radiation therapy. JVIR 1997; 8: 781- 88.
81. Rosch J, Bedell J, Puttnam J, Antonovic R, Uchida B. Gianturco expandable wire stents in the treatment of superior vena cava syndrome recurring after maximum- tolerance radiation. Cancer 1987; 60: 1243-46.
82. Rodriguez VI, Njo KH, Karim AB. Hypofractionated radiation therapy in the treatment of superior vena cava syndrome .Cancer 1993; 10: 221-28.
83. Perez CA, Presant CA, Van amburg AL. Management of superior vena cava syndrome. Semin. Oncol. 1978; 5: 123-34.
84. Boumghar M. Superior vena cava compression syndrome. Analysis of three observations of surgical decompression. Ann. Chir: Chir. Thorac. Cardio-vasc. 1985; 39: 507-11.

85. Straka C,Ying J,Kong FM,Willey CD,Kaminski J,Kim N.Review of evolving etiologies, implications and treatment strategies for the superior vena cava syndrome. Straka et al. SpringlerPlus (2016); 5 :229.
86. Yedlicka JW, Schultz K, Moncada R, Flisak M. CT findings in superior vena cava obstruction. Semin Roentgenol 1989; 24: 84-9.
87. Dhaliwal RS, Das D, Luthra S, Singh J, Mehta S, Singh H. Management of superior vena cava syndrome by internal jugular to femoral vein bypass. Ann Thorac Surg 2006; 82:310-312.
88. Lochridge SK, Knibbe WP, Doty DB. Obstruction of the superior vena cava. Surgery 1979; 85: 14-24.
89. Ampil FL, Caldito G, Devarakonda S, Vora M, Mills G, and Milligan S. Longevity after radiotherapy of stage III lung cancer: superior vena cava obstruction is associated with early mortality. Ann Palliat Med 2018; 7(2):242-248.
90. Wang J, Liang J, Wang W, Ouyang H, and Wang L . Malignant thrombosis of the superior vena cava caused by non-small-cell lung cancer treated with radiation and erlotinib: a case with complete and prolonged response over 3 years. Onco Targets Ther. 2013; 6: 749-753.
91. Büstgens FA, Loose R, Ficker JH, Wucherer M, Uder M, Adamus R. Stent Implantation for Superior Vena Cava Syndrome of Malignant Cause. Rofo. 2017 May; 189(5):423-430.
92. Marcy PY, Magne N, Bentolila F, Drouillard J, and Bruneton JN, Descamps B. Superior vena cava obstruction: is stenting necessary? Support Care Cancer 2001; 9:103-107.
93. Kim HJ, Kim HS, Chung SH. CT diagnosis of superior vena cava syndrome: importance of collateral vessels. AJR Am J Roentgenol 1993; 161:539-42.
94. Putila J, Guo NL.Combining COPD with clinical, pathological and demographic information refines prognosis and treatment response prediction of non-small cell lung cancer.PLos One 2014; 9(6):e100994.
95. Kim H, Lussier YA, Noh OK, Li H, Oh YT, Heo J. Prognostic implication of pulmonary function at the beginning of postoperative radiotherapy in non-small cell lung cancer. Radiother Oncol 2014; 113(3):374-8.
96. Martins SJ, Pereira JR.Clinical factors and prognosis in non-small cell lung cancer. Am Clin Oncol 1999; 22:453.
97. National Comprehensive Cancer Network.NCCN Clinical Practice Guidelines in Oncology v.1.2016.Non-Small Cell Lung Cancer. Available at: http://.nccn.org/professionals/physician-gls/pdf/nscl.pdf.
98. Reck M, Popat S, Reinmuth N, Ruysscher D, Kerr KM, Peters S, ESMO Guidelines Working Group. Metastatic non-small-cell cancer (NSCLC): ESMO

Clinical Practice Guidelines for diagnosis, treatment and follow-up. Ann Oncol 2014; 25 Suppl 3:27-39.
99. Tjulandin S,Imyanitov E,Moiseyenko V,Ponomarenko D,Gurina L,Koroleva I,et al.Prospective cohort study of clinical characteristics and management patterns for patients with non-small lung cancer in the Russian Federation:EPICLIN-lung.Curr Med Res Opin 2015;31(6):1117-27.
100. Mose S, Stabik C, Eberlein K, Ramm U, Böttcher HD, Budischewski K. Retrospective analysis of the superior vena cava syndrome in irradiated cancer patients. Anticancer Res. 2006 Nov-Dec;26(6C):4933-6.

SUMMARY

Bronchopulmonary cancer (PBC) is the main cause of superior venous syndrome (SSS). The aim of this study is to establish a clinical, radiological and evolutionary profile of SCS associated with PBC, to examine the modalities of therapeutic management, and to evaluate survival while identifying and analysing prognostic factors.

This is a retrospective study of patients followed for SCS secondary to primary bronchopulmonary cancer. In 41.7% of cases, SCS was the first presenting sign of the neoplasia, while 16.6% of cases presented with SCS metachronously. The histological type most frequently associated with SCS was small cell lung carcinoma (40.7%).

Contrast-enhanced thoracic computed tomography (CT) is the key examination for the diagnosis of SCS. The most common CT finding was tumour invasion of the superior vena cava (62.2%). Short-term prognosis depends on the consequences of cerebral and laryngeal oedema and associated complications, while long-term prognosis is mainly influenced by the underlying aetiology.

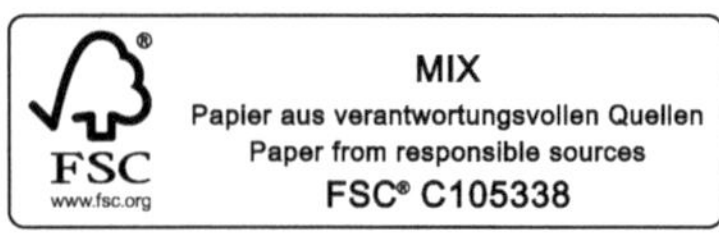

Printed by Books on Demand GmbH, Norderstedt / Germany